crewsNajafi

THE MYOFASCIAL RELEASE MANUAL

Carol J. Manheim, MSc, PT
Diane K. Lavett, PhD

SLACK Incorporated, 6900 Grove Road, Thorofare, New Jersey 08086

Editorial Director: Cheryl D. Willoughby
Publisher: Harry C. Benson

Copyright ©1989 by SLACK Incorporated

All rights reserved. No part of this book may be reproduced, stored in a retrieval system or transmitted in any form or by any means, electronic, mechanical, photocopying, recording or otherwise, without written permission from the publisher, except for brief quotations embodied in critical articles and reviews.

Manheim, Carol J.
    The myofascial release manual / Carol J. Manheim, Diane K. Lavett.
        p.   cm.
    Includes bibliographical references and index.
    ISBN 1-55642-108-7 (pbk.)
    1. Manipulation (Therapeutics) 2. Stretch (Physiology) 3. Physical therapy. I. Lavett, Diane K. II. Title.
    [DNLM: 1. Fascia—physiology. 2. Muscles—physiology. 3. Physical Therapy—methods. 4. Relaxation Techniques. WB 545 M277m]
    RM724.M34 1992
    615.8′2—dc20
    DNLM/DLC
    for Library of Congress   92-20555

Printed in the United States of America

Published by: SLACK Incorporated
              6900 Grove Road
              Thorofare, NJ 08086-9447

Last digit is print number: 10   9   8   7   6   5

Authors

Carol J. Manheim, M.Sc., P.T.
12 Carriage Lane
Charleston, South Carolina

and

Diane K. Lavett, Ph.D.
Department of Biological Sciences
SUNY Cortland
Cortland, New York

For the ease of those who read
The Myofascial Release Manual, male gender pronouns have been used.
We regret there are no concise or appropriate
unisex terms that could have been used.
The invention of these is awaited with impatience.

Acknowledgments

Portions of this book previously appeared in *Myofascial Release: A Nontraditional Approach To Stretching*, published by Forum Medicum in the Postgraduate Advances in Physical Therapy Continuing Education Course II, under the sponsorship of the American Physical Therapy Association.

The authors acknowledge Richard C. Soltys for innumerable hours of library work and the Department of Biological Sciences, SUNY Cortland, for general support. Both Ron Kaplan and Paul Kaplan assisted in the preparation of the early drafts of this manuscript. Our photographer, Michael Whittemore, through his artistic vision, was able to demonstrate muscle structure being stretched in minute detail. Patti Bagg, P.T., made helpful suggestions throughout the preparation of this book and assisted with the photography. Annie Ruth Wright also helped at every stage in the preparation of this book.

Contents

Introduction

Myofascial release, or myofascial stretching as some call it, differs from other stretching techniques in a very basic manner. Myofascial stretching relies entirely upon the feedback received by the therapist from the patient nonverbally through the patient's tissues. Although myofascial release is commonly presented as a technique that the patient controls through feedback from his body, the locus of control is the therapist who must correctly interpret and respond to the feedback. It is the therapist who determines how much, how long and how forceful the stretching will be, according to responses of the patient's body.

The determination of appropriateness of treatment is not a conscious or left brain function, but rather is transmitted entirely in a right brain manner through the sensation of touch. When the therapist responds to the proprioceptive feedback from the patient, the therapist will find that the direction of stretch, the amount of force, and the duration of the stretch is quite different from when the therapist was using any other technique of stretching. Often, very specific restrictions in the soft tissues will be found, as revealed by the line of pull, which would never have been addressed when using another stretching technique.

In order for the therapist to use the techniques described in this manual successfully, the therapist will have to make the following assumptions. First, the techniques of myofascial stretching work even though the exact mechanism of how they work has yet to be elucidated. Second, by utilizing the feedback received from the patient's body, the therapist can effectively stretch restricted structures in a manner more comfortable to the patient than can be done with traditional stretching techniques; this can be done without sacrificing the effectiveness of the stretch. Third, stretching in this manner removes restrictions that impede efficient movement. Fourth, myofascial stretching is a very safe technique and there is no danger that the therapist will inadvertently over-stretch the soft tissues of the body when the techniques are being applied properly.

By requiring the therapist to respond to the subtle changes that occur in tissue tension during myofascial stretching, the therapist is able to work with the patient and not on the patient. This is a very different philosophic base from that which is taught in many other techniques. This philosophic stance takes the therapist out of the role of expert or god-like figure and places him on an even plane with the patient. The patient participates as an equal in the treatment process. Thus, stretching of restricted tissues which impede efficient movement does not become a power play between the therapist and the patient. Instead, the philosophic orientation of myofascial stretching promotes patient cooperation and enlists the active participation of the patient in the healing process.

The therapist who is learning myofascial stretching should realize that, in order to make maximal use of these techniques the natural body rhythm, called the craniosacral rhythm by Upledger,[1] needs to be integrated as part of patient feedback. It is this rhythm, in addition to the direct proprioceptive feedback from the tissues being stretched, which dictates to the therapist the direction of pull, the amount of force, and the duration for which the force is applied. A full discussion of the craniosacral rhythm is outside the scope of this book. Thus, what is being presented is myofascial stretching without the craniosacral component. Despite this omission, the beginner can use myofascial stretching with full confidence that over-stretching and too vigorous stretching will not occur. At a later time, the student can add to his knowledge and effectiveness by exploring the craniosacral rhythm. This information is available in Upledger and Vredevoogd[1] and Manheim and Lavett.[2,3]

Myofascial release leads to postural and alignment changes. Therefore, the effects of myofascial stretching are measured by an assessment of body alignment and overall posture. The ultimate goal of myofascial stretching is optimal body alignment, which allows for the most efficient use of energy for daily tasks. The philosophy in myofascial treatment is to treat all malalignments which predispose the patient to future injury, whereas in other systems of treatment the adage is "if it isn't broken, don't fix it." Thus, the key is prevention of future injury while dealing with the current problem for which the patient is being treated.

Soft tissue injuries, while widely diagnosed as strains, sprains, or inflammation, receive minimal attention in the education of most physicians. Soft tissue injury falls between the cracks of the medical specialities. For this reason, the patient with soft tissue injury may be seen by a general practitioner, an internist, an orthopedic surgeon, a neurologist, or a rheumatologist. Unfortunately for the patient, medical treatment may mask the pain while leaving soft tissue restrictions which can continue to cause dysfunction, if not pain. Too often the medical community falls into the trap of treating the pain and not treating the dysfunction. When both the pain and dysfunction are treated simultaneously, the recurrence of problems is less likely.[4]

How many times do we hear that we, as therapists, are the first medical professionals to place our hands on the patient's body to palpate the soft tissues? How many times do we hear that we are the first to examine the patient's ability to move? How many times do we hear that we are the first to listen to the patient's story in an effort to assess the nature of the injury? How many times do we hear that we are the first to confirm that patients have, in fact, a physical problem and not a problem that is "all in their heads"?

As therapists, we must let our education and sensitive hands guide us in the treatment of our patients. Our treatments need to be directed and mediated by the information we gain from our patients verbally and nonverbally, through touch. If we do not touch, do not sense through touch the pain of our patients and do not let this pain determine our treatment, then our patients will continue to suffer from pain and dysfunction, and they will be prevented from recovering as fully as possible.

As therapists, we are uniquely qualified to address the problems of soft tissue injury and treatment. We have learned to see under the skin with our fingers. We have learned to detect dysfunction that other medical professionals may not see because they rely on visual inspection and x-rays, neither of which can reveal the true nature of soft tissue dysfunction.

Myofascial release is a very powerful technique which allows us to treat soft tissue dysfunction that does not respond to other methods. As with any method of treatment, myofascial stretching should not be used exclusively. It is another method of approach, an adjunctive treatment which gives us still another weapon in our arsenal, allowing us to remove the spectra of pain from our patient's bodies.

Many therapists have been using soft tissue mobilization methods for years without actually referring to it as such. The philosophic difference between soft tissue mobilization and myofascial release lies in permitting and encouraging the patients to be equal participants in the process of removing restrictions from their bodies. As a therapist becomes skilled in this technique, patient feedback becomes very consistent and positive. Comments such as: "How did you know that's where I hurt?" "That's exactly where it hurt when I twisted my ankle" or "I had forgotten about that. How did you know it was there?" occur repeatedly. Once the therapist begins receiving this type of feedback, there will be no question that myofascial release as a technique is accurate, useful, and effective.

The purpose of this book is to teach the technique of myofascial stretching as a mechanical skill. Once the student has learned the skill, then he needs to learn how and when to use this skill. Therefore, I have left the evaluation process to the end, so as not to confuse the student while learning the skill. Likewise, trigger-point releases and balancing the dural tube are also left to the end. The transition of this mechanical technique into a therapeutic art is the intangible change to which all therapists must aspire. Art is the difference between therapists and their effectiveness in applying these principles of treatment. This change comes with practice of the skill and with the application of the "people skills" we all use.

An Overview of Treatment

First, the area to be stretched is palpated to determine the area of restriction. Next, the tissues are stretched gently along the direction of the line of the muscle fibers until a resistance to further stretch is felt. This stretch position is held until the soft tissues are felt to relax. The relaxation is due to the dissipation of a restriction and is called a "release." It is sensed by the therapist and the patient as a "softening" or "letting go."[1] Then, the tissues are stretched further to take up the slack created by the release and are held in this new elongated position. The process is repeated until the tissues are in a fully elongated position or until no further stretching can be tolerated. The above describes the essence of myofascial release; the rest of this discussion is commentary.

An "emotional release" may occur at any time during a myofascial release, a trigger point release, during massage, or as a response in general to the physical contact required by myofascial release. When an emotional reaction is triggered by physical contact, it is called a "somato-emotional" release.[1] Somato-emotional release, which sometimes is also called "full body unwinding," is a large and complex topic and outside the scope of this lesson.[5-7] For a detailed discussion of somato-emotional release, see Upledger and Vredevoogd[1] and Manheim and Lavett.[2,3] Suffice to say, should an emotional release occur, the therapist needs to be open and accepting of whatever the patient says.

Myofascial Restriction and the Anatomy of Fascia

Myofascial restrictions can be visualized in several different ways. Each gives a conceptual model on which to base the evaluation and treatment of patients using myofascial release. Imagine all of the fascia in the body to be a continuous air-filled balloon with bubbles which are attached to it and which house the various organs and muscles. If part of the balloon is distorted by tightness or restriction, then all parts of the balloon must be distorted to compensate. The smallest tug or pull will be felt throughout the balloon just as the smallest puff of wind will change its direction of movement.

Alternatively, consider all the fascia in the body to be a square of plastic wrap. If the plastic wrap is pinched or is stuck on itself, the sheet can no longer be a square and will no longer cover the entire body unless the body twists and folds to fit under the altered shape of the sheet. The sheet must be smoothed out again to fulfill its function in an efficient manner.

Picture a skeleton with tight red plastic overlays depicting the muscles and fascia. As the overlays are stretched, they change to white along the lines of stress. For example, place the latissimus dorsi on the right side of the skeleton and the quadratus lumborum on the left. Fully flex the right humerus, retract the right shoulder, and protract the right side of the pelvis. The left side of the pelvis must then be retracted and the lumbar spine must rotate. Picture the stress lines in the quadratus lumborum as the left side of the body is rotated to the right. Pick any two other muscles and place them on the skeleton instead. Put one of the muscles on its maximum stretch, then visualize the resultant stress on the other muscle. This game can be played over and over with the same result each time, showing that any myofascial restriction at, near, or far from a target muscle causes distortions not only in the target muscle, but in other muscles as well. Thus, all myofascial restrictions must be treated and released to restore proper alignment and energy-efficient movement to the entire system.

Fascia has been regarded as extraneous tissue without consideration that it might have a distinct function all its own. As Garfin et al. state,[8] "The functional relationships between fascia and the forces and pressures generated by the underlying muscular contractions are poorly understood." Few research projects have studied the biomechanical effects of fascia on muscle or explored the effect that removal of the fascia has on the underlying muscle and osseofascial compartment.[8] In the medical model, when severe fascial restriction occurs, the fascia is removed without consideration of any additional biomechanical consequences the loss of fascia might produce. In fact, fascia assists in maintaining muscular force by controlling muscle pressure and volume, and the effect of fasciotomy is a 15% loss of muscle strength.[8] Myofascial release, an alternative to removal, is frequently capable of decreasing myofascial constriction and the accompanying pain, which is diagnosed as compartment syndrome, without compromising muscle strength.

Few anatomy texts show fascia other than as a structure to be removed to expose the more important organ systems. Cailliet, in contrast, lists fascia as a type of connective tissue along with tendons, ligaments, cartilage, muscle and bone.[4] In a schematic drawing of fascia, the fascia is actually divided into three layers. The first is a superficial layer that contains fat, nerve endings, and blood vessels. The second layer is called a potential space. This space may enlarge with extravasation or edema, suggesting that the fascia can be disrupted and stretched by any injury, no matter how minor. The third layer is the deep, investing layer and below that lie layers of other tissue, such as pleura, peritoneum, and pericardium. Individual muscle groups are enveloped by fascia separating one muscle group from the next. Fluid between the fibers of the fascia acts as a lubricant, allowing free movement of one muscle past another. Bursae are formed in some areas between muscles, between muscle and tendon or bone, or beneath the skin over bony prominences. Septa extend from the outer fascial layers into the muscle. These septa divide the muscle into progressively smaller units, ultimately surrounding each myofibril.[4,9,10]

The connective tissue fibers that form the fascia are arranged approximately in one plane to form membranes. The fibers run in various directions so that they appear interwoven with no one direction predominating. This is in contrast to tendons, in which fibers run roughly parallel to each other.[9] Because the fibers in fascia run in all directions, they allow the fascia to be distensible in all directions to accommodate changes in muscle bulk and to be stretched. Fascia shrinks when it is inflamed. It is slow to heal because of a poor blood supply and it is a focus of pain because of its rich nerve supply.[4]

General Instructions for Myofascial Releases

To learn the following techniques, you must be relaxed and able to focus entirely on the feedback coming through your hands. I always work in a darkened room, ask my patients to close their eyes, and close my eyes also. In addition, I ask my patients to let their minds wander and stay non-focused. You should also have your eyes closed and a clear mind, attending only to the sensations under your hands. As you relax and the patient relaxes, you will feel the inherent tissue motion under your hands. The reason for closing your eyes is to let your hands be your eyes. We are so used to letting what we see override what we feel that this technique cannot be learned with your eyes open. You cannot see feelings. You need to focus on what you are feeling, which should be the feedback that you are getting from your patients, so that you can respond to that feedback. The patients need to close their eyes to block out distracting stimuli and allow total focus upon the sensations within their own bodies. This will allow the patients to relax maximally and become aware of physical tension that is helping to maintain a restriction.

Stretching a Single Myofascial Group

Any muscle that allows the placement of two hands or even two fingers can be gently stretched to relieve myofascial restrictions. Hand placement should be comfortable for both you and the patient. For a large muscle group such as the erector spinae (Fig. 1), the middle trapezii (Fig. 2), or the quadriceps femoris (Fig. 3), you may gain better leverage by crossing your hands. For a small muscle like the masseter, only one or two fingers are needed with uncrossed hands (Fig. 4).

Place each hand or finger proximal to the attachments of the muscles to be stretched, using just enough pressure to stretch the superficial skin and fascia and to stretch the underlying muscle(s) in the direction of the muscle fibers. This should be done in a firm manner. Hold this position until all the soft tissue is felt to relax, then stretch again, taking up the additional slack created by the release. Repeat this process until no further stretch is possible and both the muscle and related soft tissues are in a fully elongated position. Slowly and gently release your stretch pressure and reevaluate for restrictions.

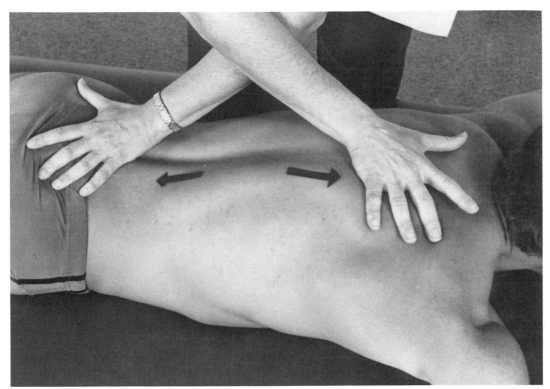

Figure 1: Cross hand longitudinal stretching of the lumbar and thoracic erector spinae muscles.

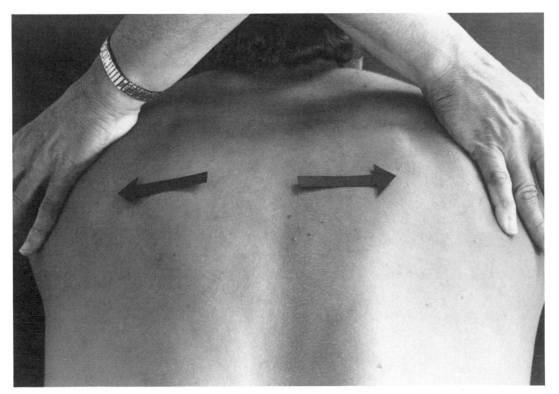

Figure 2: Cross hand longitudinal stretching of the middle trapezii muscles.

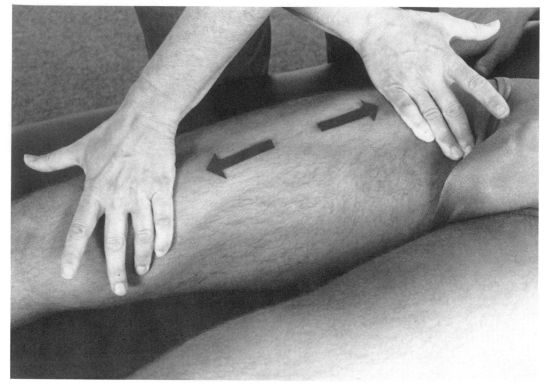

Figure 3: Cross hand stretching of the quadriceps femoris muscle.

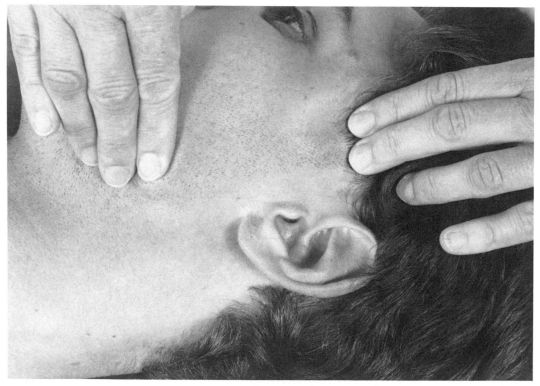

Figure 4: Stretching the masseter muscle using two fingers of each hand.

Fascia of the Arm and Shoulder Regions

The superficial fascia of the arm and shoulder contain a variable amount of fat. Superficial nerves and blood vessels run through both the superficial and deep fascia. The tough membranous layer of brachial fascia encloses the muscles of the arm, forming a sheath completely around the arm. This sheath is loose fitting anteriorly to allow bulging with muscle contraction. Posteriorly, the fascia is fused to the flatter triceps brachii muscle. Medially and laterally, the fascia is attached to the humerus, forming the medial and lateral intermuscular septa.[9,10]

In addition to containing a variable amount of fat, the superficial fascia in the pectoral region encloses the glandular breast tissue. The superficial fascia is not well developed in this region and is most often fused with the deep fascia. The fascia divides and splits to surround each structure in the pectoral region and then reunites to form a single layer again. It is attached to the bony prominences and also gives attachment to some of the fibers of the underlying muscles. Each muscle has its own fascial coat.[9,10]

Releases in the Arm and Shoulder Region: The Arm Pull

Stand next to your patient's hip. Your patient's forearm should be supinated. Hold onto your patient's hand gently, with one hand holding the hypothenar eminence and the other hand holding the thenar eminence, in a comfortable manner. Do not hold with your fingertips, but use your thenar eminence to hold onto the hand, gently spreading the patient's palm and reversing the usual concave posture of the palm (Fig. 5). During the arm pull, stretch the interosseous muscles and the palmar fascia at the same time you stretch the entire upper quarter during the arm pull. Many patients will give you very positive feedback to this specific hand grip. It feels very good to have the palm stretched, releasing tension that is rarely recognized or felt until the contrast of relaxation is felt. There is also a large psychological component to the firm and long-term contact of hand on hand, going back to our youngest days when holding an adult's hand meant security and safety.

Move toward your patient's feet so that you are in position to place traction on the arm, pulling downward towards the feet in line with the fibers of the deltoid muscles (Fig. 6). You must be in a comfortable position to be able to remain relaxed and not become tired. Those of you who are tall may need to bend your knees to avoid stressing your lower back, or you may choose to sit on the edge of the plinth or on a stool. Those of you who are short may be uncomfortable reaching slightly upward and may wish to use the same positioning strategies of sitting on the edge of the plinth or sitting on a high stool or you may want to stand on a riser or stool. Do whatever is needed to position yourself for comfort and for efficient movement.

Put a gentle amount of traction, approximately five pounds, on the arm. Maintain the traction, focusing on how the hand and arm feel, and wait for the soft tissues to relax. As they relax you will feel a gentle give of the entire arm. Apply a little more traction to take up the slack and wait again for a release to occur. Continue doing this until an "end feel," the sensation of no further stretching being available, has been reached. This indicates that the arm is stretched as far as it can be in that position at that time.

Once you have reached that point, ask your patient to cross his legs. What happened to what you were feeling? Most of the time this will give you an immediate sensation of more tension in the system or even a sensation of twisting in the system. Sometimes a release will occur with this movement of the legs, not necessarily from actually crossing the legs, but rather from the shift of focus and the deep breath taken as the movement is performed.

Now have the patient tense his crossed legs and feel again how much more tension is present in the arm you are holding.

Next, have your patient tighten up the crossed legs and then relax them. Feel the increase followed by a decrease in tension flowing through your hands.

Have your patient relax and uncross his legs. Now tense up your arms and shoulders and let them relax. What did that do? Tension in you will override what you are feeling from your patients. Therefore, you have to stay relaxed while you are doing this or you throw "noise" into the system.

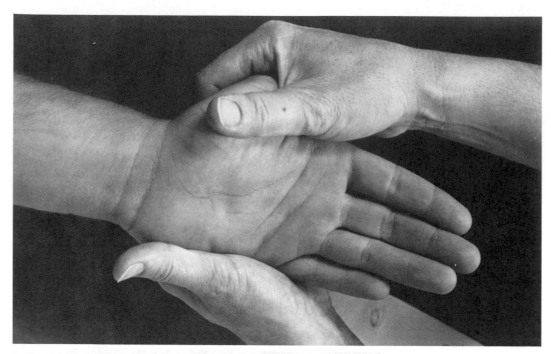

Figure 5: Stretching of the interossei muscles by gripping the hand on the thenar and the hypothenar eminences. As the palm is stretched laterally, the normal concave posture will flatten. Using your fingers as a fulcrum on the back of the hand, add a slight backwards force ending with the palm in a slightly convex posture. As with all releases, this should be done slowly to allow the tissues to respond.

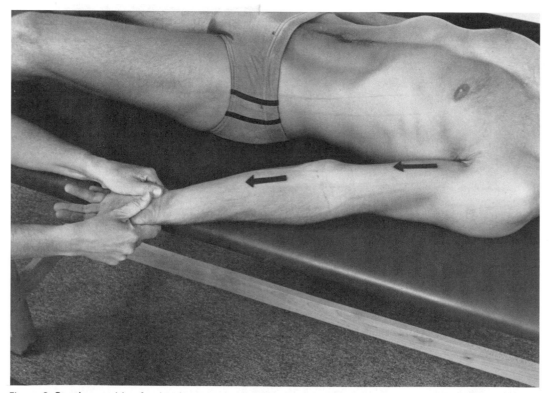

Figure 6: Starting position for the single arm pull. Begin the arm pull with patient's arm at his side, in external rotation, so that his thumb points to the direction of movement. Apply traction in line with the longitudinal arm musculature and in line with the fibers of the deltoid muscles.

At this point, with the arm stretched as far as the soft tissues will allow, visualize with which muscles you have been primarily dealing. You should see that it is the deltoid muscles that we have been keying in on from the line of pull, along with all the muscles in the hand, forearm, and upper arm.

Now, very slowly and gradually come out into abduction (Fig. 7), maintaining the entire arm in external (lateral) rotation. As you do that, part of the range of motion is going to feel like you have just "grooved in." This is a feel of smoothness and rightness of position. Everything feels to be in balance. You will recognize the sensation the first time you feel it. When you hit that point, pause, wait for a release, and then continue slowly leading the arm into more abduction if the arm is not already starting to lead you into that position. The arm may begin to move spontaneously at any point in the range of motion. If that occurs, follow the motion placing just enough tension on the arm to keep the movements slow. This will allow you to feel hesitations or restrictions. When one is felt, stop the motion and wait for a release before allowing the motion to continue.

If you have a patient with a pathological condition around the shoulder joint, in the anterior chest wall, or in the parascapular region, you will reach a point at which it just does not feel right to continue. Back off a few degrees, stop, and wait for the releases that allow you to continue. This is done entirely on the patient feedback you are getting through your hands. If the verbal feedback from your patient does not coincide with what you are feeling, trust your feelings and respond to them. You cannot have a preconceived idea of how far the range of motion is going to go or of how much progress you are going to achieve at any given time. If no further releases occur, then the flexion portion of this maneuver is completed and you will need to move into horizontal adduction and scapular protraction as described below.

Bring the arm around into full abduction until the elbow is proximal to the ear (Fig. 8). Continue the circle by bringing the arm across the body from this position, rolling your patient onto his side. As your patient rolls, grasp your patient's hand with your right hand. Bring your left hand down to the

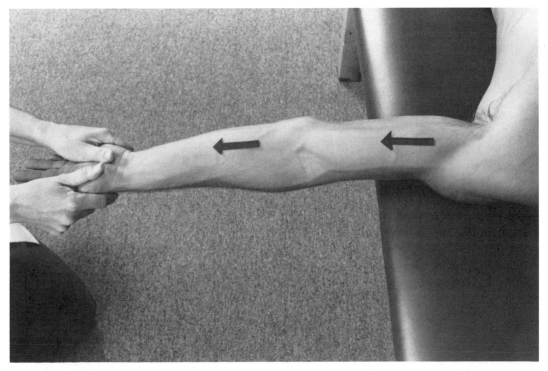

Figure 7: Moving into abduction during the single arm pull. If the arm does not spontaneously move into abduction, gently and slowly abduct the arm, while maintaining traction and continuing the arm pull. As tightness or hesitations are felt, stop the motion, maintain the traction, and wait for the tissues to relax before continuing the abduction. Do not allow the motion to continue through any tightness.

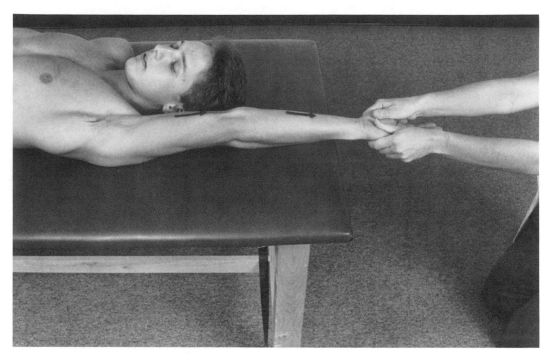

Figure 8: Stretching to full abduction during the single arm pull. Continue to follow the spontaneous movement or move the arm further into abduction until the arm is next to the ear. If your patient does not have full range of motion at the shoulder joint, you may need to allow the arm to flex at the shoulder joint while abducting. The final position will be abduction with flexion. It is not functionally necessary to achieve pure abduction without flexion.

scapula, hooking around the medial border of the scapula and distracting the scapula (Fig. 9). Let the patient's arm lead you around. Bring the arm forward in complete protraction. As the scapula is distracted outwardly, you will feel it release and ride forward on the rib cage until it is as far forward as it will go.

Once you have the scapula fully distracted, bring the arm into internal (medial) rotation and reverse the circle (Fig. 10). Again, move slowly and feel for any hesitation. When you feel hesitation, hold and wait for it to relax before you continue. If it feels as if the arm wants to pull backward, put some compression into the shoulder joint (Fig. 11). Wait for the relaxation and then distract again. Be sure, as your patient rolls onto his back, that he does not leave his legs crossed. Most will be so relaxed at this point that their legs will automatically cross as they resume the supine position from the side-lying position

The arm pull is not a technique "written in stone" with definite hand grips that must be followed to achieve maximal results. The heart of this technique is responding to patient feedback, as felt through your hands. If you have a patient who, for some reason, does not permit you to hold his hand, you can shift your grip to above the wrist (Fig. 12) to the mid-forearm (Figs. 13-14) or to above the elbow (Fig. 15). You can use any hand-hold that is comfortable to you and to your patient and that achieves the objective that you and your patient set for that treatment session. Please always keep in mind that the objective is often set and achieved in totally nonverbal communication.

While doing an arm pull, trigger points can be treated as they are found in the soft tissues at any point in the range of motion, if the trigger points are preventing full elongation of the muscle. Thus, changing the hand-hold is sometimes necessary to release trigger points and also to direct the release of other restricted tissues that are preventing full range. Because of trigger point releases, you may find yourself placing one hand on the pectoral muscles (Fig. 16) to encourage their relaxation at one point in the range and on the latissimus dorsi muscles during another point (Fig. 17). The knowledge of where to place your hands always comes from feedback from the patient's body. Until you achieve

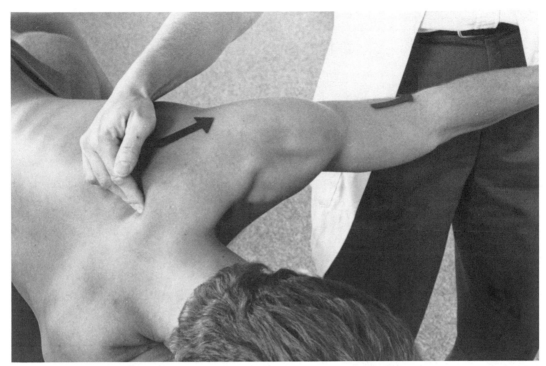

Figure 9: Stretching to full horizontal adduction during the single arm pull. Once full abduction is achieved in the frontal plane, continue to follow or lead the arm into horizontal adduction across the patient's body, while distracting and protracting the scapula. Throughout this motion, the arm continues to be externally rotated so that the thumb points to the direction of movement.

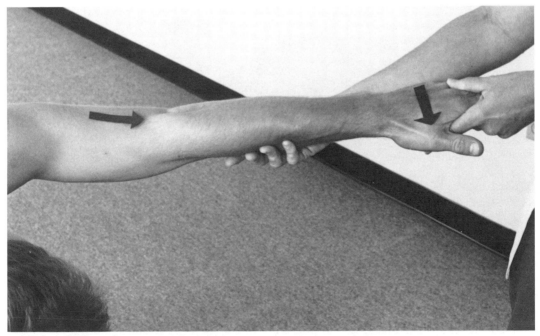

Figure 10: Reversed single arm pull. Once full distraction of the scapula is achieved and all muscles are relaxed, slowly place the arm into internal rotation. Be alert to any hesitations or tightness and wait for the muscles of external rotation to relax and stretch. Once again, the thumb is pointing toward the direction the arm is moving. Slowly retrace the circle of movement until the arm is once again adducted to the patient's side but in internal rotation.

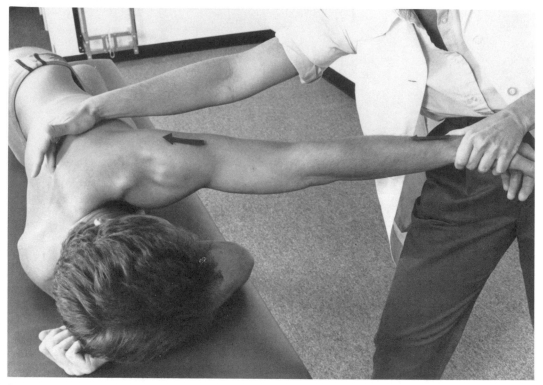

Figure 11: Compression of the shoulder joint in response to scapular retraction.

A. If the shoulder begins to retract spontaneously, compress the shoulder joint and retract the scapula by pushing the arm back into the joint and releasing your distraction at the medial edge of the scapula. When relaxation of the scapular retractors occurs, resume traction on the arm and protraction of the scapula.

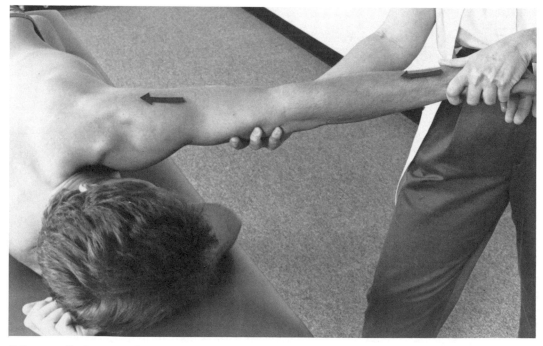

B. If your patient cannot tolerate compression of the elbow joint at the same time, you may want to shift your hand to just above the elbow instead.

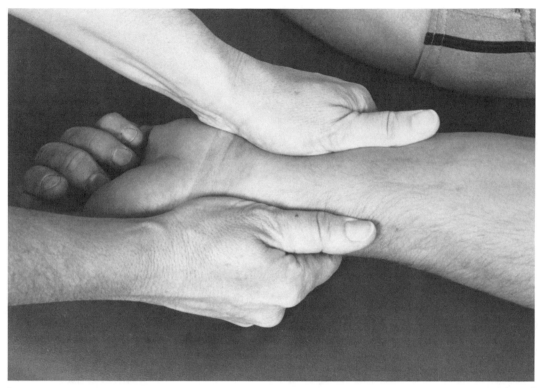

Figure 12: Alternate hand placement for the arm pull, holding above the wrist. If the patient complains of wrist or hand pain during the arm pull, he will be unable to relax and allow full stretching of the upper quarter. The pronator quadratus muscle can be stretched at the same time with this grip.

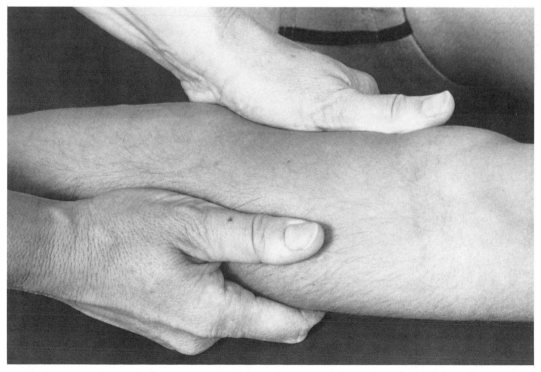

Figure 13: Alternate hand placement for the arm pull; holding in the upper portion of the forearm. The pronator teres muscle can be stretched at the same time with this grip.

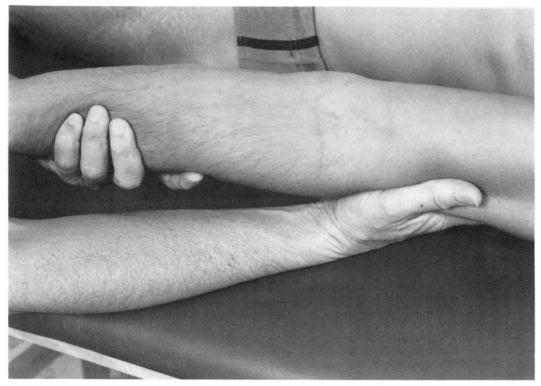

Figure 14: Alternate hand placement for the arm pull, holding above and below the elbow.

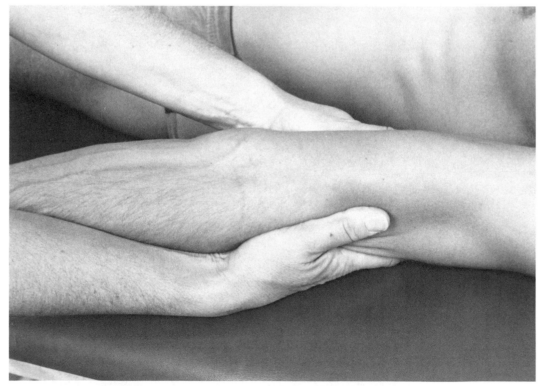

Figure 15: Alternate hand placement for the arm pull, holding above the elbow.

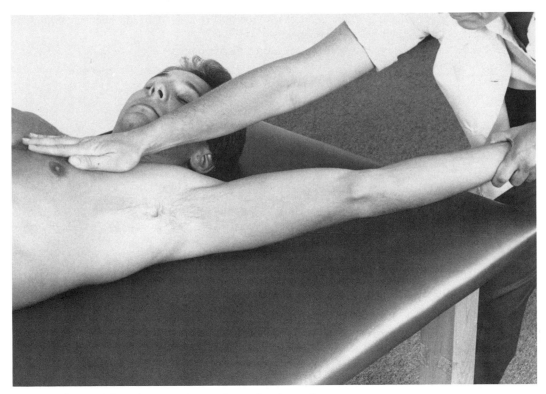

Figure 16: Arm pull focusing attention on the pectoral muscles.

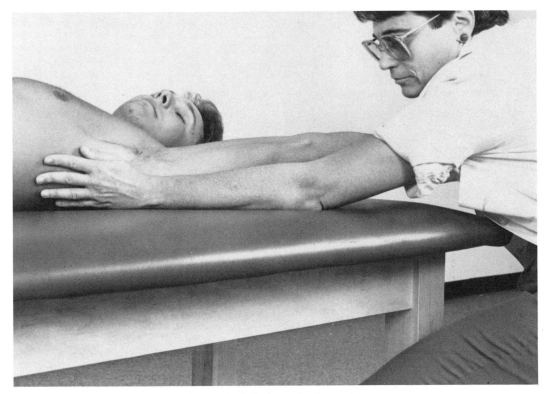

Figure 17: Arm pull focusing attention on the latissimus dorsi muscle.

the sensitivity and confidence to allow feedback to guide you, you can follow the above directions and your patient will still gain significant benefits.

A discussion of trigger points and the release of these points is found on pages 75-80. It is important to learn the technique of myofascial stretching first, before adding trigger point releases into the basic technique. Trigger points may be released during the process of myofascial stretching and may not require later specific attention. Thus, maximum stretching should be achieved at all points in the range of motion before any trigger point releases are attempted.

Fascia of the Lower Extremities

The fascia of the lower extremities is extremely well developed. The fascia lata encloses the posterior hip musculature and the muscles of the thigh. The fascia lata is especially strong on the lateral border of the thigh where it includes the longitudinal iliotibial band. Strong intermuscular septa extend on each side of the quadriceps femoris muscle, attaching to the femur. Medially, septa border the adductor canal which houses the femoral artery as it extends into the popliteal space. Cylindrical fascia enclose the lower leg musculature with septa on each side of the peroneal muscles attaching to the fibula. A transverse septum separates the deep and superficial calf muscles. The lower leg fascia holds the tendons that pass from the leg to the foot, where well developed fascia exist on the dorsum and in the sole of the foot.[9,10]

The Leg Pull

With the patient in the supine position, gently cup the heel in one hand while dorsiflexing the foot with the other hand and maintaining the hip in full extension (Fig. 18). While holding the foot in a neutral position, place approximately five pounds of traction on the leg and wait for the release to occur. Once the initial release has occurred, gently increase your traction by taking up the slack. Again, wait for the release. Continue to do this until an end feel is achieved. At the end point, no further relaxation will occur and the leg will feel to be as fully extended as possible.

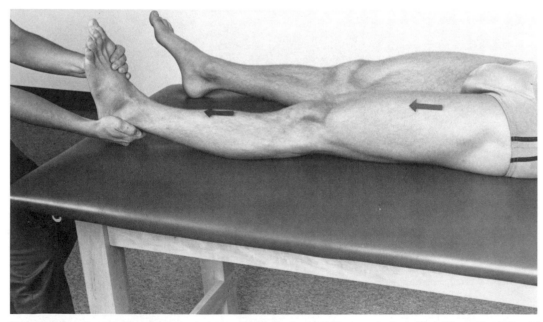

Figure 18: Starting position for a single-leg pull with the foot held in a neutral position. The patient should not be actively dorsiflexing the foot to neutral, but should be held in neutral by the therapist. As equal traction is applied, symmetrical relaxation should occur. If the relaxation is not symmetrical, then adjust the traction in response to the feedback from your patient's body.

Now, gently externally rotate the leg as far as your patient can permit while maintaining the hip and knee in full extension (Fig. 19). If full external rotation is not immediately achieved, repeat the process of externally rotating the leg until tightness is felt; back off a few degrees, hold until a release occurs, take up the slack and again, wait. Traction must be maintained throughout this process.

Once full available external rotation is achieved, if the leg has not already begun to abduct, gently move the leg into abduction (Fig. 20). Move the leg slowly so that you feel any hesitation or tightness in the range of motion. At the point of hesitation or tightness, stop, back up a few degrees, and hold that position until a release is felt. Then, continue to abduct through the available range. Once again, maintain the distraction of the hip throughout this maneuver.

When full abduction is achieved in the sagittal plane, allow flexion to begin at the patient's hip to complete the circle (Fig. 21), allowing the leg to cross over the midline of the body (Fig. 22). As your patient rolls onto his side, continue distracting the leg to stretch the gluteal and the piriformis muscles fully. At this point, the leg may try to come down into full extension again or it may tend to go into further hip flexion. If the leg begins to move spontaneously, follow the motion while maintaining just enough tension on the lower extremity to keep the motion slow. When a restriction or hesitation is felt, stop the motion and hold until a release occurs.

Once you have achieved a full stretch of the leg and hip musculature with your patient still on his side, move his foot to place the hip into internal rotation (Fig. 23). Repeat the release process until full internal rotation is achieved, and then reverse your motion. If the hip pulls back into retraction, compress the hip joint by pushing the leg into the hip joint (Fig. 24). As relaxation occurs, resume the traction. Continue the circle back with the leg internally rotated, allowing your patient to roll onto his back until the leg is once again adducted with full hip and knee extension (Fig. 25).

If your patient has a pathological condition at the hip joint, full range of motion may not be achieved. Should spontaneous movement occur, there is no need to continue through the full leg pull because the patient will be showing you which restrictions need treatment. Because you are responding to patient feedback through your hands, you will not exceed the safe range of motion for your patient. If your patient cannot tolerate the pressure of your hand at the ankle (Fig. 26) or dorsiflexion of the ankle (Fig. 27), any alternate hand grip or position may be used that is mutually acceptable (Fig. 28).

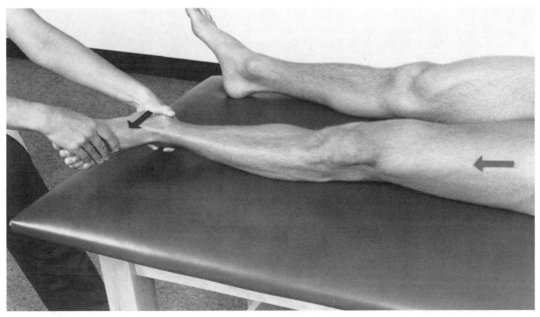

Figure 19: Stretching into external rotation during a single-leg pull. While maintaining traction, slowly move the foot and leg into external rotation, waiting for any tightness of the internal rotators to release and permit full range of motion.

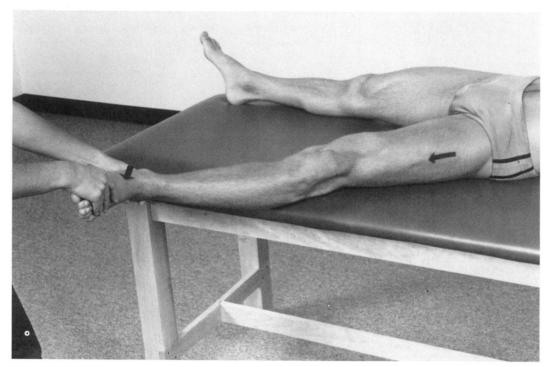

Figure 20: Abduction and external rotation during a single-leg pull. Once maximum external rotation and traction are achieved, bring the leg slowly and gently into abduction if spontaneous abduction does not begin. Follow or guide the leg to full abduction, repeating the same movement with the leg as was described with the arm.

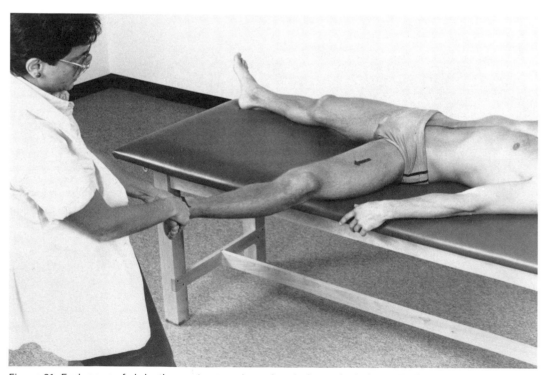

Figure 21: End range of abduction and external rotation during a single-leg pull. The amount of abduction available will vary greatly from patient to patient. It is only through the proprioceptive feedback from your patient that you will know when the maximum is reached.

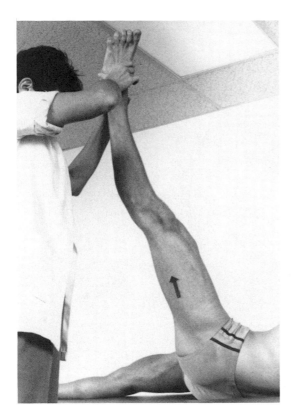

Figure 22: Horizontal adduction, external rotation, and protraction at the midrange of a single-leg pull. When full abduction is reached, guide the leg into horizontal adduction while maintaining traction on the leg. This will bring the pelvis into protraction as the hip is both flexed and adducted to 90 degrees.

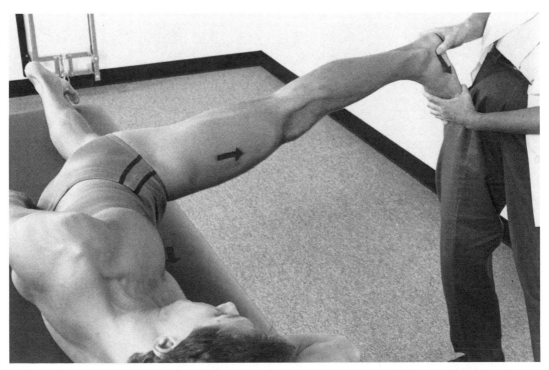

Figure 23: Beginning of the reverse single-leg pull with the leg adducted and internally rotated. When full horizontal adduction is complete, slowly place the leg into internal rotation, waiting for any tightness to be released before proceeding. Retrace the arc of motion, releasing any tightness as it is located until the leg is back in the starting position.

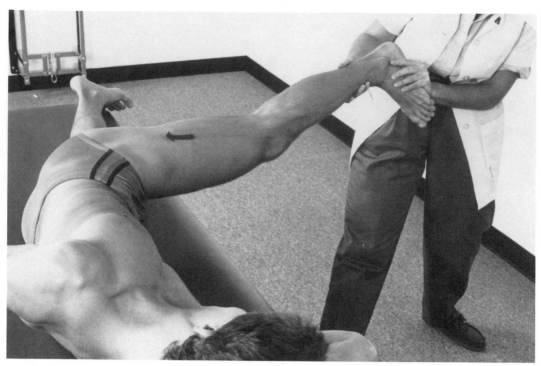

Figure 24: Compression into the hip during the reverse single-leg pull. If the pelvis begins to retract, compress the hip joint in the same manner as you would the shoulder joint, wait for the release and resume traction again.

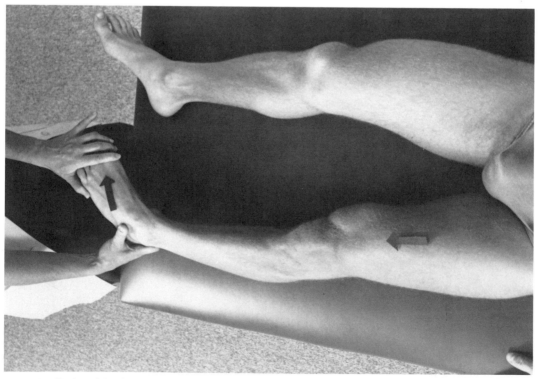

Figure 25: End position for the reverse single-leg pull. Note that the model has very limited internal rotation at the end range. Forefoot adduction will occur giving the impression of internal rotation.

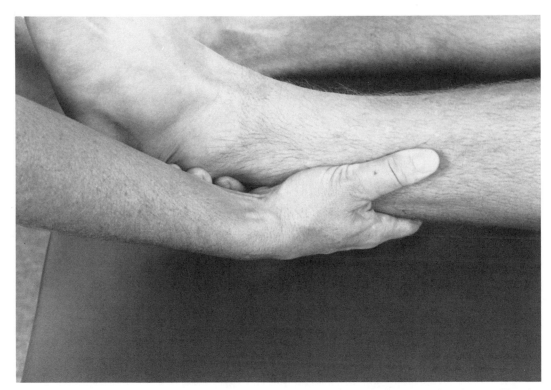

Figure 26: Alternate hand grip for a single-leg pull with one hand above the ankle and the other cradling the calcaneous.

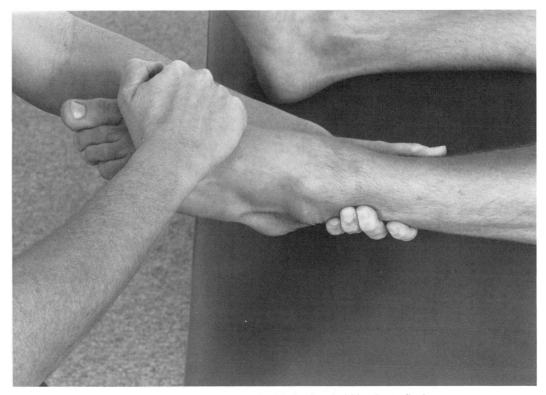

Figure 27: Alternate hand grip for a single-leg pull with the foot held in plantarflexion.

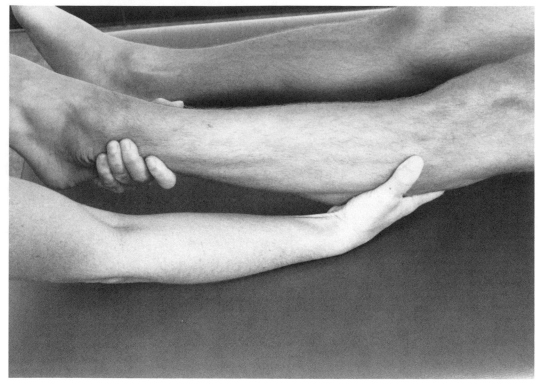

Figure 28: Alternate hand grip for a single-leg pull with the hands widely spaced on the lower leg avoiding traction on the ankle joint.

Stretching the Iliopsoas Muscle

Tightness of the iliopsoas muscle results in an increased lordotic curve and flexion at one or both hip joints. Care must be taken to prevent a compensation to substitute for true stretching. For example, if the pelvis is not prevented from tilting, hip extension may appear to be increasing when, in fact, the lordotic curve is increasing instead.

The iliopsoas muscle presents an unique problem when using myofascial release techniques. All the other muscle groups have allowed direct access to at least some of the muscles being stretched; direct pressure could be applied which would guide the direction of stretch. In contrast, all portions of the iliopsoas are inaccessible to gentle touch so that direct feedback cannot be gained from the muscle. The entire technique must be considered to be indirect; the feedback is transmitted through the leg and is muted by the distance it must travel.

Position the patient in the supine position with his target buttock at the edge, or even over the edge, of the plinth (Fig. 29). For comfort of the patient and stability, the other leg may be flexed at the hip and knee. Keep a steadying hand on the ilium, trying to maintain neutral rotation. Allow the knee to flex to ninety degrees and extend the thigh over the edge of the plinth. The thigh will be in abduction in addition to extension. Place your other hand either on the mid-thigh or at the knee and gently take up any available slack in the muscle by traction downward (Fig. 30). Observe the low back and prevent compensation through hyperextension of the lumbar spine by fixing the ilium in a neutral position. If hyperextension does occur with the ilium held in neutral, move the thigh back into hip flexion until the spine is in its usual lordotic position or until the lordotic curve is flattened.

Once the optimal position for the low back is found, try to maintain this while stretching the iliopsoas and the other muscles which flex the hip joint. Using the upper leg as the lever and the ilium as the fulcrum, stretch the iliopsoas while keeping the pelvis in a neutral position. Wait for the release and stretch again. Because the feedback is very dilute, extra care must be taken not to overpower the muscle rather than waiting for the releases to occur.

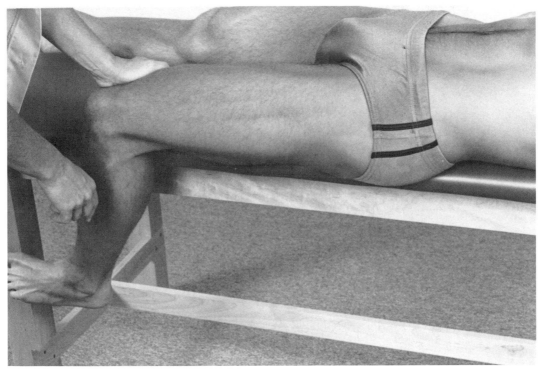

Figure 29: Patient position for stretching the iliopsoas muscle with the buttock over the edge of the plinth and the knee flexed.

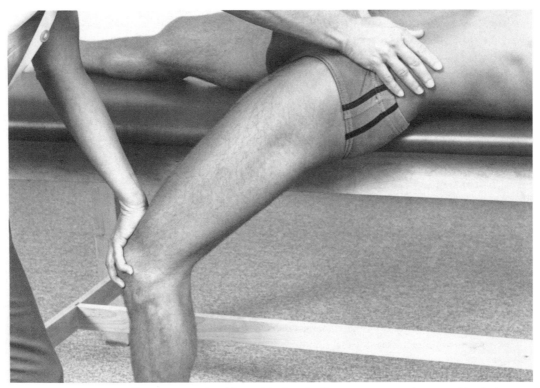

Figure 30: Stretching the iliopsoas muscle with one hand on the ilium to prevent an increased lordotic curve substituting for hip extension, and the other hand at the knee using the leg as the lever.

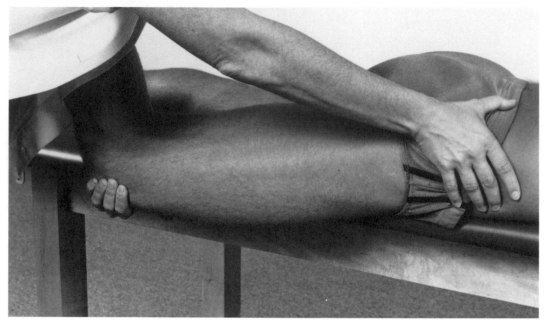

Figure 31: Prone position with the pelvis over the edge of the plinth for stretching of the iliopsoas muscle. This position cannot be used with the patient who has bilateral hip flexion contractures which prevent him from lying flat. Bilateral flexion contractures place the low back into an exaggerated lordosis with the prone position.

The supine position is the position of choice if the patient has significant hip flexion contractures which prevent him from lying flat in the prone position. However, the iliopsoas and the other hip flexor muscles can also be stretched with the patient prone and the hip flexed over the side of the plinth (Fig. 31). This position will allow somewhat greater control over the lordotic curve because gravity will assist in holding the pelvis in a neutral position. The counter pressure can be placed on the posterior rim of the pelvis, spreading the pressure out more evenly. The major disadvantage of this position is that the therapist must support the full weight of the leg, in addition to overcoming the force of gravity.

Stretching the Piriformis Muscle

Special attention is often paid to the the piriformis muscle when the patient's major complaint is pain radiating along the innervation path of the sciatic nerve. Excess tension in this muscle can mechanically compress the sciatic nerve, no matter whether it passes over the top, goes through, or passes under the piriformis. Once again, we are dealing with a muscle that cannot be palpated directly and the feedback is diluted by the leg being used as a lever.

To stretch the piriformis muscle, the patient is supine with the contralateral leg extended. The leg to be stretched is flexed at the hip and knee, with the foot resting on the lateral border of the contralateral leg (Fig. 32). The thigh is in neutral rotation and adduction. The piriformis muscle is stretched by moving the leg into more adduction, internal rotation, and hip flexion.

The Cervical Fascia

The prevertebral fascia continues laterally from the front of the cervical vertebrae, covering the longus colli and the scalene muscles, and extending dorsally into the fascia covering the levator scapulae muscles. Fascia extends between the muscles and attaches to the cervical vertebrae. Inferiorly, the fascia extends to the outer borders of the thorax. The space between the middle and prevertebral fascia forms the visceral compartment that houses the larynx, trachea, esophagus, thyroid gland, brachial plexus, and subclavian artery.[9,10]

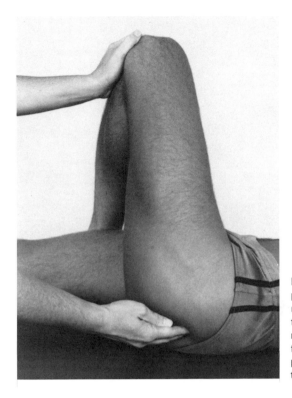

Figure 32: Supine position for stretching the piriformis muscle. As the piriformis muscle relaxes, the knee is moved closer to the contralateral shoulder while the thigh is internally rotated and adducted. Pressure is placed on the fibers of the piriformis as they are exposed by this position. This also encourages relaxation through a simple feedback loop.

Stretching the Posterior Cervical Musculature

Ask your patient to remove all jewelry prior to stretching of the posterior cervical musculature. Gently palpate the carotid pulse one side at a time since simultaneous palpation can provoke a carotid reflex (Fig. 33). The pulses should be roughly equal in strength.[11] A significant difference in the strength of these pulses or vertebral artery disease are definite contraindications for any vigorous movement of the head and neck. Test for vertebral artery disease by fully rotating the neck in both directions, holding in the extreme range for a few seconds (Fig. 34), or by placing the neck into hyperextension (Fig. 35). Observe the patient's pupils for dilatation while doing this. The patient with vertebral artery disease will complain of vision disturbances and light headedness with neck rotation and with neck hyperextension.[12] Before any extensive myofascial stretching of the neck, shoulders, or head, a thoracic inlet release should be performed (see below).

Position yourself comfortably at your patient's head, place your hands gently on your patient's shoulders, and have your patient move down far enough so that you can keep your elbows fully supported on the plinth while cradling his skull in your hands (Fig. 36). Now, gently cup both hands around the base of the skull and place approximately five pounds of traction on the posterior cervical musculature, pulling the head into extension by stretching the short neck extensors (Figs. 37-39).

Complaints of radiating pain are common with this maneuver, secondary to active or latent myofascial trigger points. It is almost impossible to avoid placing pressure on these trigger points during this stretching procedure. As relaxation is achieved, the radiation pattern should decrease or disappear entirely, depending on the sensitivity of the trigger points. It may be necessary to perform trigger point releases during stretching of the posterior musculature. A description of trigger point releasing is found on pages 76-80.

Maintain traction at the base of the skull until a release is felt and then gently increase traction to take up the slack. This will progressively pull the head into extension, further decreasing the cervical lordotic curve. If the patient tries to move into hyperextension, indicating very tight short neck extensors, ease back on the amount of traction until his head is again in capital extension. Then, reapply traction until you just barely feel resistance and hold in that position until the release is

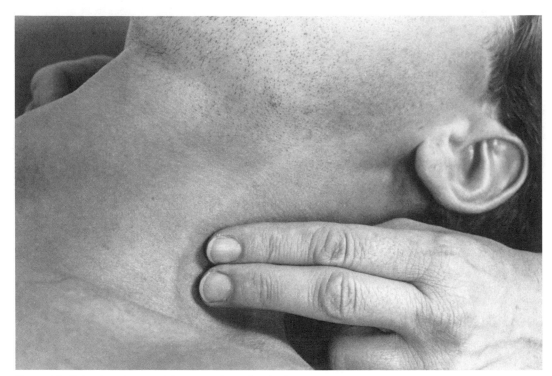

Figure 33: Palpating the carotid artery prior to beginning treatment, with the head in a neutral position.

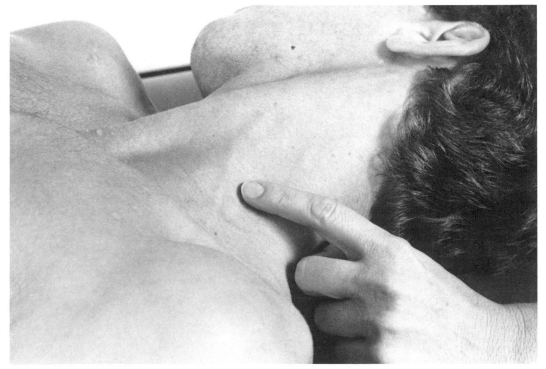

Figure 34: Palpating the carotid artery prior to beginning treatment, with the head in lateral rotation.

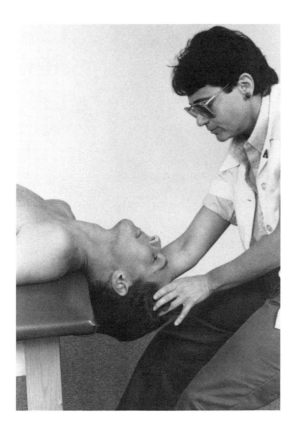

Figure 35: Palpating the carotid artery prior to beginning treatment, with the head in hyperextension. Observe the patient's pupils in this position also. The pupils should contract in response to the light.

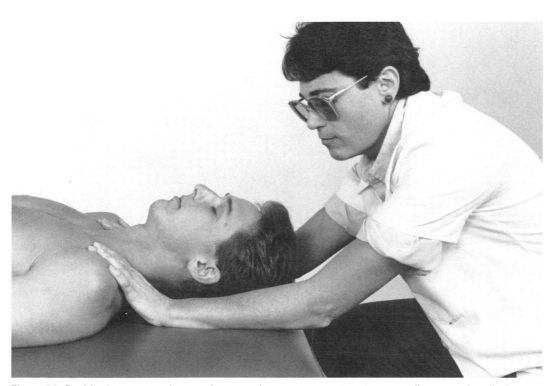

Figure 36: Positioning your patient to give you adequate room to support your elbows on the plinth.

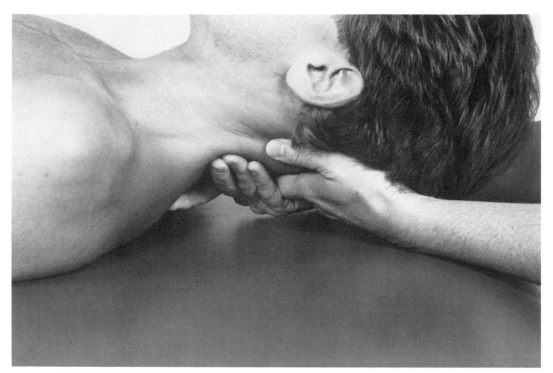

Figure 37: Beginning position for stretching of the posterior cervical musculature.

A. Stroke the posterior cervical musculature several times in long sweeping strokes before placing both hands at the base of the occiput.

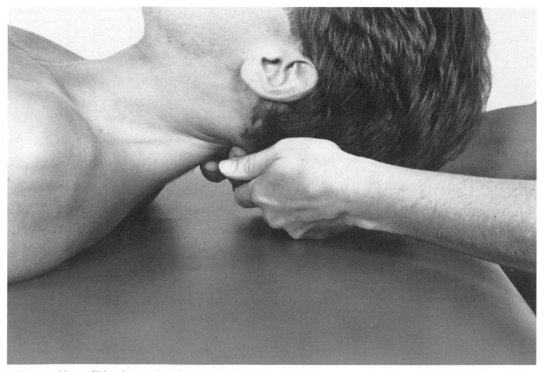

B. The stroking will begin to relax the muscles and will also help set your hands properly at the base of the occiput.

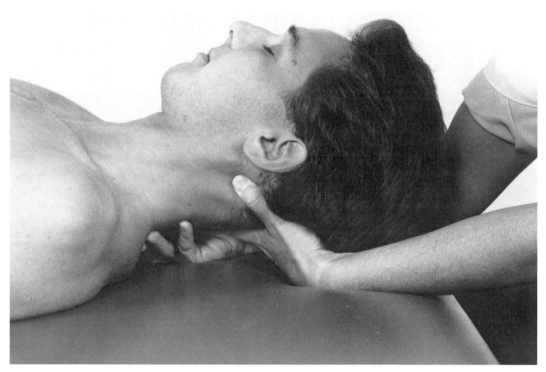

Figure 38: Alternate hand placement for stretching of the posterior cervical musculature, with one hand at the base of the occiput and the other at the base of the neck.

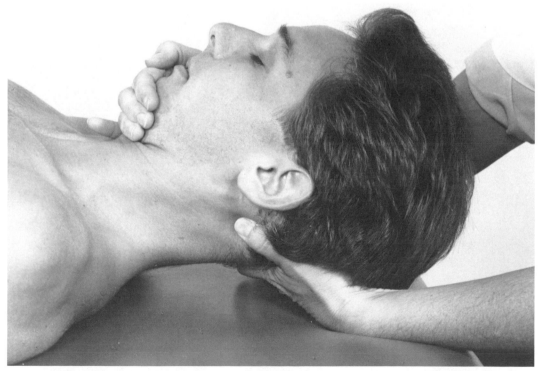

Figure 39: Alternate hand placement for stretching of the posterior cervical musculature, with one hand at the base of the occiput and the other at the chin. With this grip, gentle pressure can be placed on the chin downward to counter a forward head posture. Note the tension in the sternocleidomastoid muscle, in addition to the tension in the posterior cervical musculature.

achieved. You may need to change your hand position to focus attention on the restriction or to provide more efficient countertraction (Fig. 40). Continue until an end feel is achieved. If your patient has difficulty relaxing in this position once you have taken up the available slack in the muscles, ease back a few degrees and ask him to take a deep breath and exhale fully several times. Often, the release will occur with exhalation.

Some patients will begin to go into spontaneous cervical movements with this amount of stimulus. The movements generally consist of lateral rotation and, occasionally, hyperextension and flexion of the neck. Should this occur, continue to follow the motion of your patient, placing enough drag on his head to keep the motion slow and controlled, while maintaining traction on the cervical musculature. This will feel quite different than an arm or leg moving spontaneously. As hesitation or restriction is felt, stop the motion until a release is achieved and then allow the motion to begin again. When a full release is achieved, your patient will stop the movements and completely relax, allowing you to take up slack in the muscles again. Patients who are under a lot of stress may spontaneously begin to go into a somato-emotional release as well. As mentioned earlier, somato-emotional release is outside of the scope of this presentation.

When no further stretching of the posterior cervical musculature is available, have your patient take several deep breaths to be sure full relaxation has been achieved, and then gently release your traction. Throughout this maneuver, your patient should be lying comfortably on the plinth with his legs in full extension and not crossed at the ankles. You may need to remind your patient to keep his legs uncrossed throughout the stretching procedure, since this is a frequently observed habit. If lower extremity extension causes too much stress on the patient's lower back, place pillows under his knees as you would for other treatments.

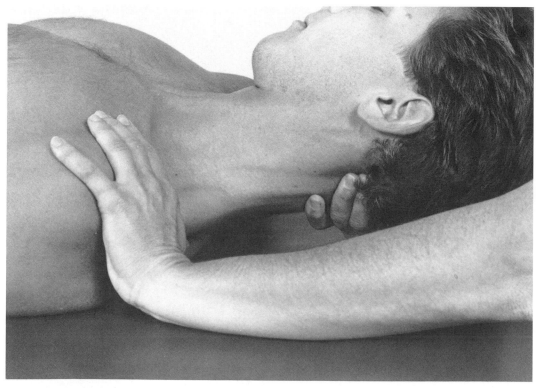

Figure 40: Alternate hand placement for stretching of the posterior cervical musculature, with one hand at the base of the occiput and the other at the lateral neck musculature.

The Cranial Base Release

When the patient's posterior cervical musculature is fully relaxed, place the palms of your hands just under the base of his skull, with your fingers extended along the neck. Now, flex your fingers at the metacarpal phalangeal joints so that you form a right angle to your palm with your fingertips at the base of the skull (Figs. 41-42). Instruct your patient to relax and to allow his head to drop into the palm of your hands. You may need to repeat this instruction several times because your patient will have the tendency to try to hold his head up off your fingertips. As progressive relaxation of the muscles that cross from the cervical region and attach to the base of the skull occurs, the head will slowly drop into your hands (Fig. 43).

Continue cradling the skull in the palms of your hands, and maintain a slight amount of traction with your second and third fingers while placing your fourth finger on the patient's first and second cervical vertebrae. Extend the fourth finger to distract the vertebrae while flexing the second and third fingers to place traction to the skull gently from the upper cervical spine (Fig. 44). When no further movement occurs, again place traction on the posterior cervical musculature, moving into the last few degrees of capital extension (Fig. 45).

This is a very sensitive area where myofascial trigger points, either active or latent, may be present. In the process of performing this release, digital pressure is placed on these trigger points and may release them as well. If these trigger points are so sensitive that your patient is unable to tolerate the amount of pressure needed to complete the release, several treatment sessions to treat the trigger points may be necessary before the cranial base is finally released.

The base of the skull is a prime area of injury during a flexion-extension injury. This common injury results in multiple trigger points. Spontaneous movement of the head and neck may occur during a cranial base release, reproducing the motions that resulted in the original myofascial injury. Should this happen, continue to follow the motion as described earlier until your patient finally relaxes and permits the cranial base release to be completed. A somato-emotional release may also be triggered in this position.

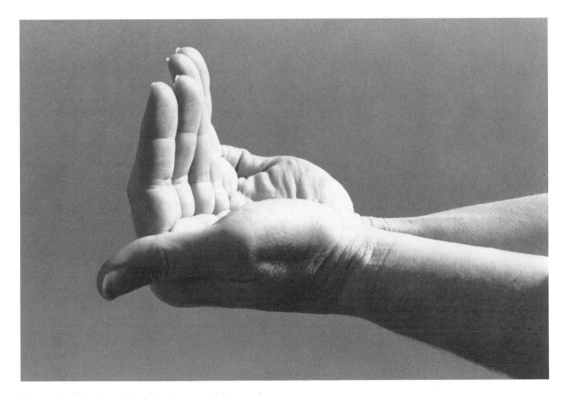

Figure 41: Hand position for the cranial base release.

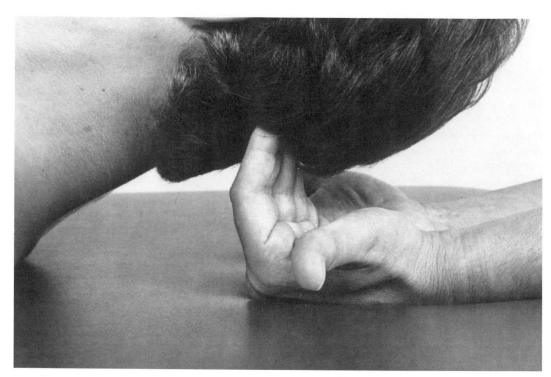

Figure 42: Beginning of cranial base release with the patient's head resting on the therapist's fingertips, placing pressure on the proximal fibers of the posterior cervical musculature. Very often, this is the site of active myofascial trigger points that cause radiating pain into the head. Some patients are initially unable to tolerate enough pressure to allow the cranial base to release. Others will talk of a good hurt and welcome the pressure.

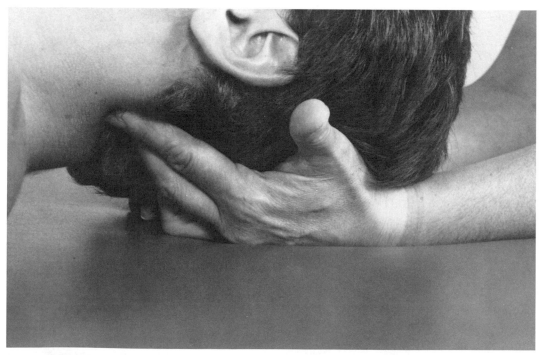

Figure 43: End of cranial base release, with the patient's head resting in the therapist's palms as the skull is being distracted from the upper cervical vertebrae.

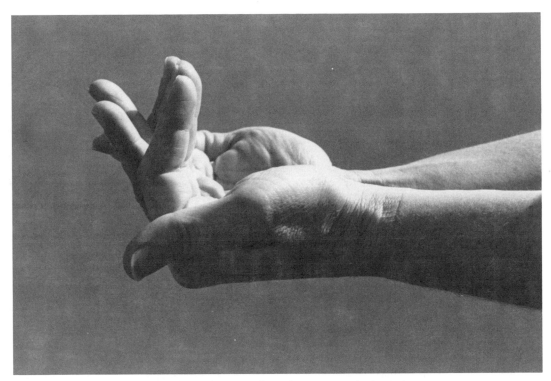

Figure 44: Hand position for distracting the skull from the upper cervical vertebrae.

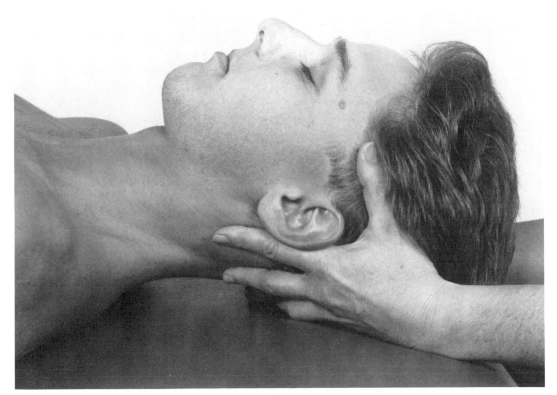

Figure 45: Final capital extension and traction following a cranial base release.

A. Note the lack of tension in the sternocleidomastoid muscle, as well as the lack of tension in the posterior cervical musculature.

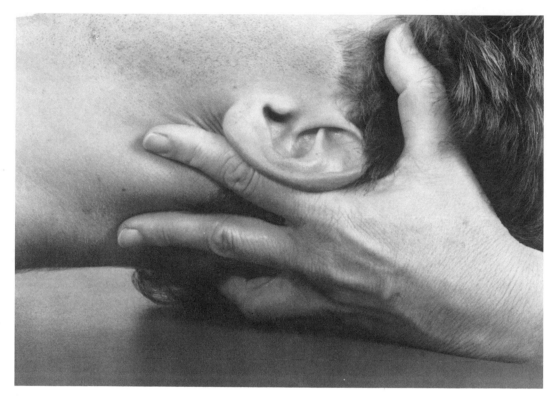

B. The head is in complete contact with the therapist's hands as the cervical lordosis is flattened. Note the distance between the neck and the plinth and compare with the distance in Fig. 39.

The Thoracic Inlet Release

Before doing any major releases above the level of the clavicle, routinely perform a thoracic inlet release. This maneuver relaxes the anterior chest wall musculature. If you are planning to stretch the posterior cervical musculature next, the best position from which to perform this release is sitting at the patient's head (Fig. 46). If you intend to stretch other muscles in the trunk or to perform an arm pull next, this maneuver can be performed sitting at the patient's side (Fig. 47).

While sitting at the patient's head, place your nondominant hand under the patient's lower cervical region and upper thoracic spine (Fig. 48), and place your dominant hand at the midline on the chest just below the sternal notch (Fig. 49). This will place your forearm and elbow along the patient's cheek. Most often, this is a very comfortable position, both for the therapist and the patient, allowing maximum contact and relaxation. This also transmits a sensation of security to the patient, and you may feel a progressive relaxation of the head and neck against your forearm during this release. Once again, instruct your patient to lie with both lower extremities extended and without crossing his legs or ankles.

Your pressure on the chest should be light to prevent direct inhibition of the inherent tissue motion. Compress the patient's body between your hands until slight resistance to your touch is felt. This is the proper amount of pressure to use. When first learning to perform the horizontal releases, you may want to ask your patient to give you feedback on the amount of pressure you are using until you are able to utilize the feedback from your hands. Once you have learned the technique, you may find you are using a heavier touch than that described earlier.

The inherent tissue motion will guide your hand in a roughly circular or oval pattern across the chest wall. At an area of restriction, the motion will cease. Continue to keep your hand in the same position with the same amount of pressure and wait. When a release is achieved, the inherent tissue motion will again begin. At a full chest wall release, you will feel a softening throughout the entire

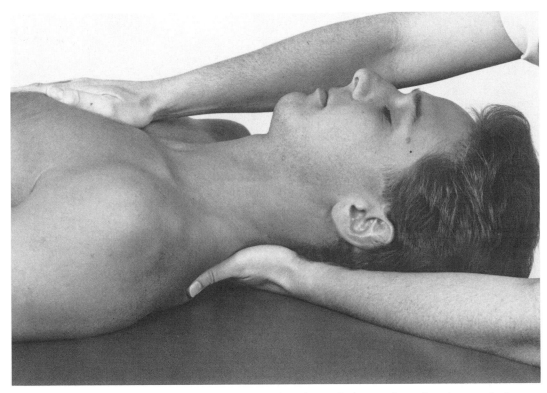

Figure 46: Hand positions for a thoracic inlet release when the cervical musculature is to be stretched next.

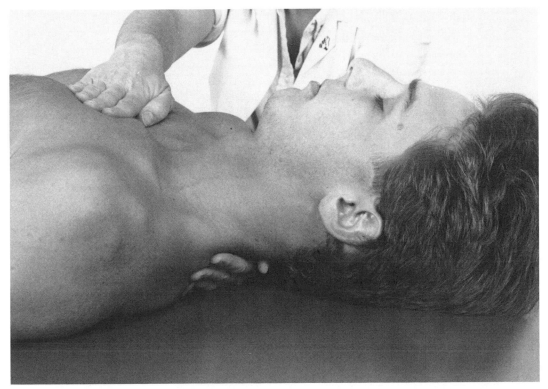

Figure 47: Side position for a thoracic inlet release when the other horizontal releases are to be performed next.

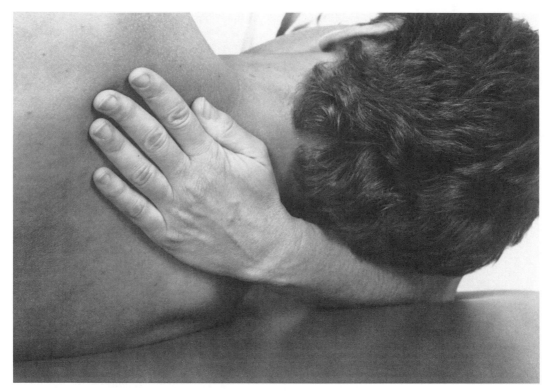

Figure 48: Hand position on the lower cervical and upper thoracic vertebrae for a thoracic inlet release performed from the side position.

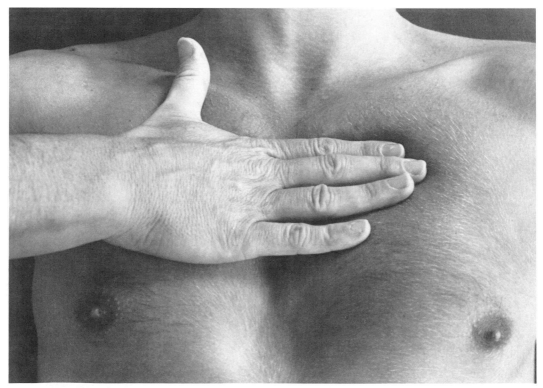

Figure 49: Hand position at the midline of the chest just below the sternal notch for a thoracic inlet release performed from the side position.

thoracic region and a profound relaxation of this area. At this point, no further relaxation is possible. It is very easy to override the patient's inherent tissue motion by using too much pressure or to lose the feel of the movement by losing your concentration. If the first occurs, lighten your touch until you feel the motion again. If the latter occurs, clear your mind of distractions and refocus your attention to the sensations under your hands.

A full release of the thoracic region is not always achieved during one treatment session. If the thoracic inlet release is being used as preparation for other stretching maneuvers, the procedure can be terminated after a partial release of the tension if no further movement is felt. If your goal of treatment is relaxation of the chest wall, however, specific stretching of the tense muscles, such as the pectoralis major, may be needed. This is then followed by another thoracic inlet release.

The Diaphragm Release

The diaphragm release is performed in the same manner as the thoracic inlet release. For this release, the therapist sits at the patient's side, perpendicular to the line of the diaphragm. While the dominant hand is placed on the patient's abdomen at the base of his rib cage (Fig. 50), the other hand is placed posteriorly on the diaphragm (Fig. 51). Once again, light pressure is used, and the hand is drawn in a circular or oval fashion, this time across the lower rib cage and abdominal region. Continue to follow the inherent tissue motion with both hands, stopping as restrictions are felt, waiting for a release, and continuing until no further restrictions are found. Remove your hands only when no further motion is felt and a feeling of relaxation is present under your hand.

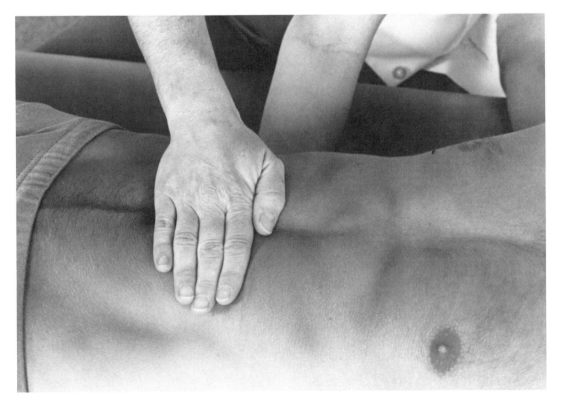

Figure 50: Hand position on the upper abdomen for the diaphragm release.

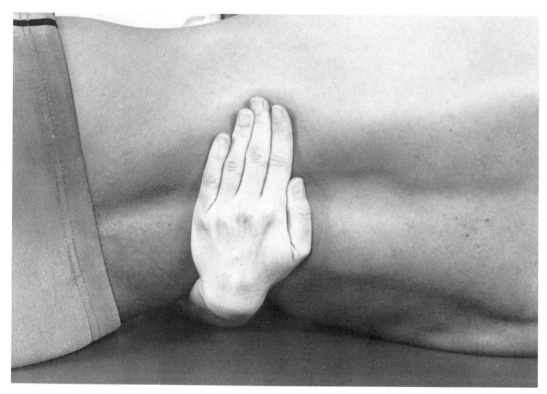

Figure 51: Hand position on the back for the diaphragm release.

The Pelvic Floor Release

The pelvic floor release is performed in the same manner as the thoracic inlet and diaphragm releases. This time, one hand is placed under the patient's coccyx (Fig. 52) with the other hand placed just above his pubis symphysis (Fig. 53). Again, a light touch is used and your hand is led around the lower abdominal wall by the inherent tissue motion. Follow the motion, releasing restrictions as described earlier, until no further restrictions are felt. When the release is achieved at the pelvic floor, often an anterior-posterior rocking of the pelvis is felt. This should be smooth, rhythmic, and symmetrical in nature. Feeling this movement is a signal that full release has been achieved.

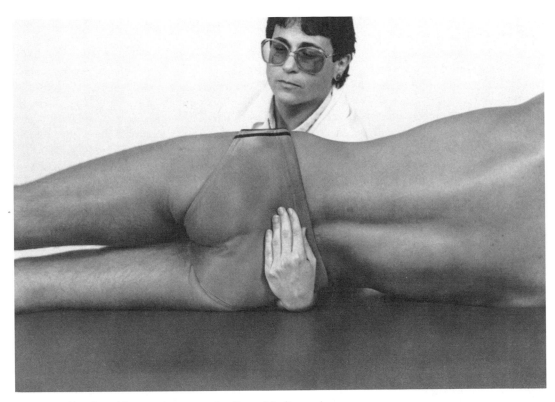

Figure 52: Hand position on the coccyx for the pelvic floor release.

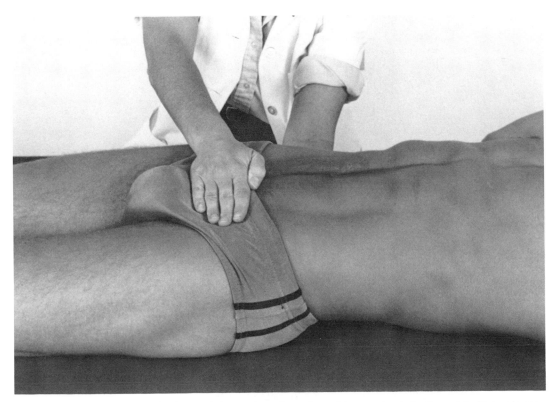

Figure 53: Hand position on the lower abdomen just above the pubis symphysis for the pelvic floor release.

The Double-Arm Pull

Depending on what other structures you want to stretch, position your patient on his back (Fig. 54) or stomach (Fig. 55) with his arms extended overhead. Grasp both of your patient's wrists with your hands. Place traction on both arms as evenly as possible, taking up the available slack. Hold this position until the soft tissues are felt to relax. Increase your traction slightly, taking up the additional slack. Repeat this process until no further stretch is possible and an end feel is reached. Slowly and gently release your traction and reevaluate for restrictions. Shoulder flexion with the patient supine will allow stretching of the shoulder girdles and the entire upper thoracic region. In contrast, the same stretch with the patient prone will allow stretching of the erector spinae muscles into an extended or hyperextended position and stretching of the anterior chest wall.

Spontaneous arm movements will rarely begin in this position. If they do begin, however, place enough traction and resistance on the arm to keep the movements slow and controlled. When restrictions are felt, stop the movement, hold until a release occurs, and take up the slack as described above.

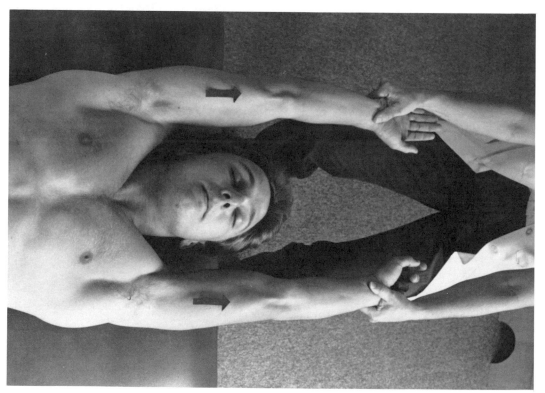

Figure 54: Supine position for the double-arm pull.

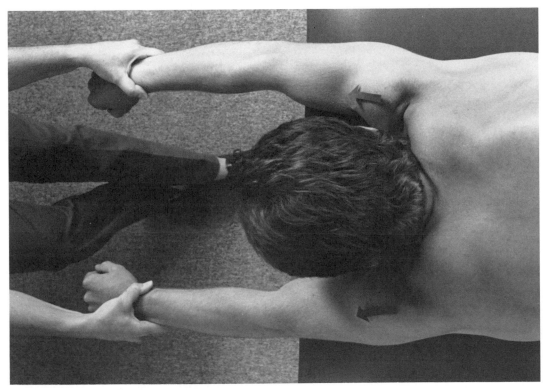

Figure 55: Prone position for the double-arm pull.

Stretching the Shoulder Portion of the Upper Trapezius Muscle

The neck portion of the upper trapezius muscle will be stretched during the procedure for stretching the posterior cervical musculature (previously described). It is also necessary to stretch the shoulder portion of the upper trapezius muscle for maximum effect.

With the patient supine, sit behind the patient's head. Place your hands gently on the upper shoulders and begin to take up the slack of the upper trapezius muscle by gently pushing downward and laterally at the same time (Fig. 56). After you have taken up the slack in the muscle, hold this position until the release is felt. With the initial release, stretch again to take up the slack and continue until an end feel is reached.

If the shoulders move independently of each other or if one side is significantly tighter than the other, it may be necessary to stretch only one shoulder at a time. In that case, position yourself over the side to be stretched if you wish to remain at your patient's head (Fig. 57). Alternatively, you may want to stand at your patient's side to get better leverage (Fig. 58).

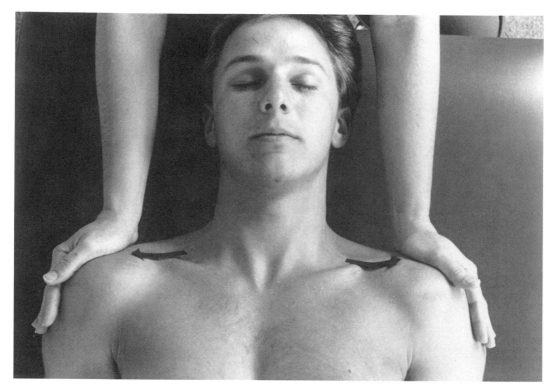

Figure 56: Bilateral stretching of the shoulder portion of the upper trapezii muscles. Note that the direction of stretch is downward and outward simultaneously.

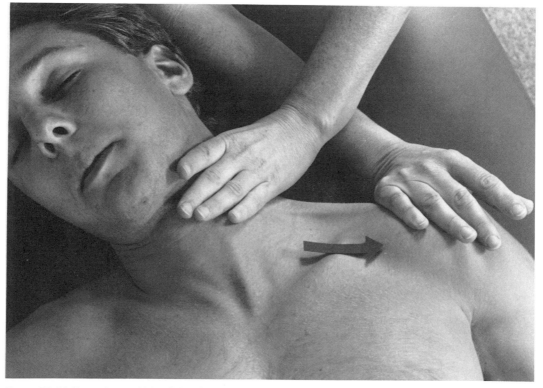

Figure 57: Unilateral stretching of the shoulder portion of the upper trapezius muscle, with the therapist at the patient's head.

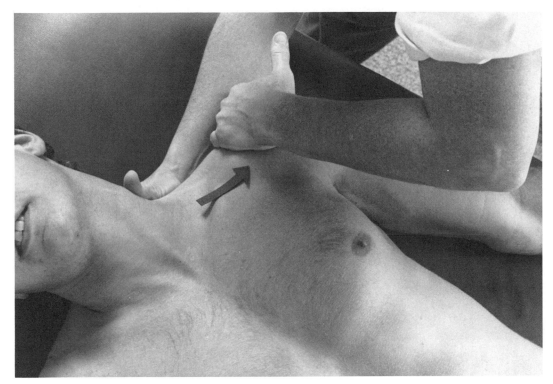

Figure 58: Unilateral stretching of the shoulder portion of the upper trapezius muscle, with the therapist at the patient's side.

Stretching the Pectoral Muscles

The pectoral muscles can be stretched from a variety of positions, depending on which muscles were stretched prior to them or what you plan to do next. The pectoralis major has two distinct portions which must be treated as different muscles for a maximum stretch to be achieved. The upper set of fibers runs parallel to the clavicle and responds to stretching in a straight lateral fashion. The lower fibers of the pectoralis major fan from the ribs and sternum up to a point where they join the tendon as it inserts into the humerus. Either portion can be stretched first.

To begin stretching the upper portion of the pectoralis major, place both hands on the muscle, gently stretching medially and laterally across the horizontal fibers (Fig. 59). When the horizontal fibers will not stretch any further, direct your attention to the fanning fibers below them (Fig. 60). Depending on where you sense restriction, you may want to move your hands down only an inch or two, taking the remainder of the muscle in very small sections.

Once the entire muscle is stretched in sequential fashion, you may want to spread your hands to cover as much of the muscle at one time as possible for a final stretch. This will tell you if any restrictions remain in the muscle and will allow you to focus your attention on any remaining myofascial restriction.

As the pectoralis major relaxes, tension in the pectoralis minor will be felt and will guide your hand placement for the optimum position to stretch it. Keep a mental image of the pectoralis minor to help direct your stretching. When no further tension is felt beneath your hand, both the pectoralis major and minor are in their fully elongated position.

Another method of stretching the pectoral muscles is by use of the arm pull, angling the arm along the direction of the fibers (Figs. 61-62). The horizontal fibers of both pectoral muscles can be stretched simultaneously in much the same position which would stretch the upper trapezii (Fig. 63). Often, you will be led to this stretch immediately following an upper trapezii stretch when dealing with bilateral protracted shoulders.

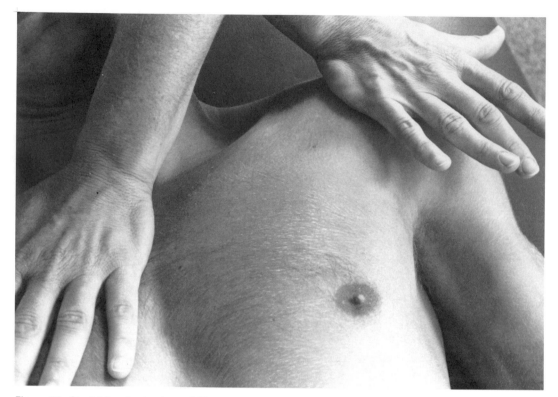

Figure 59: Stretching the horizontal fibers of the pectoralis major muscle.

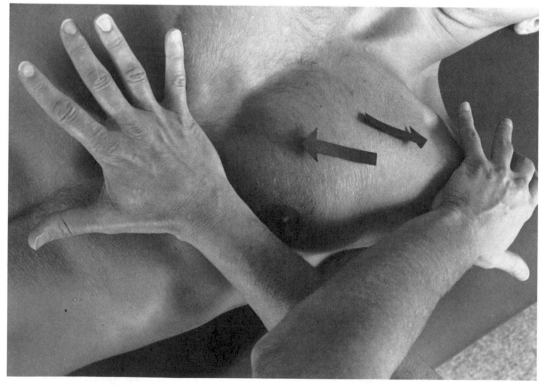

Figure 60: Stretching the lower fibers of the pectoralis major muscle.

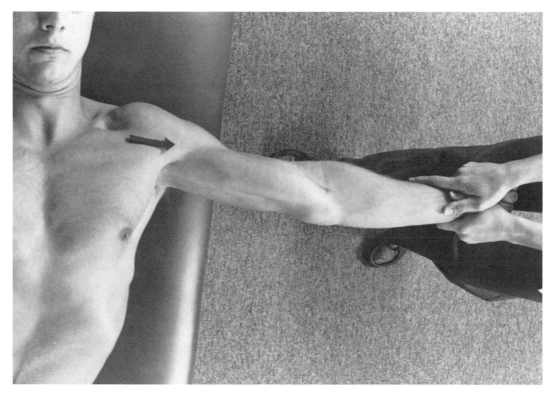

Figure 61: Stretching the horizontal fibers of the pectoralis major muscle while performing an arm pull.

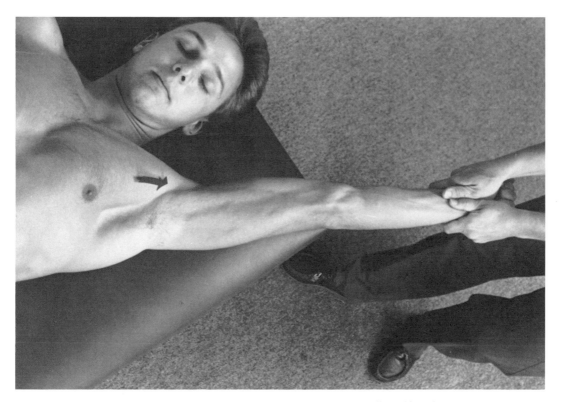

Figure 62: Stretching the lower fibers of the pectoralis major muscle while performing an arm pull.

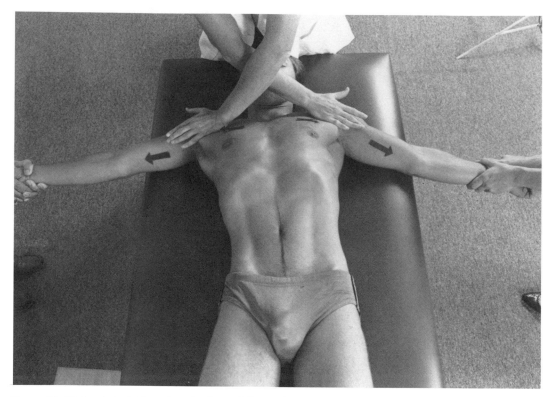

Figure 63: Bilateral stretching of the horizontal fibers of the pectoralis major muscles, with direct stretching and with bilateral arm pulls.

The Bilateral Leg Pull

With the patient in the supine position, cup both of his heels in your hands and gently apply traction to both legs, taking up the available slack (Fig. 64). As described earlier, hold the elongated position until a release occurs. Repeat this maneuver until no further stretch is possible and an end feel is reached. This maneuver will allow stretching to be achieved throughout the erector spinae muscles in the low back and the quadratus lumborum muscles. If this stretch is performed with the patient in the prone position, stretching of the hip extensors can also be accomplished (Fig. 65).

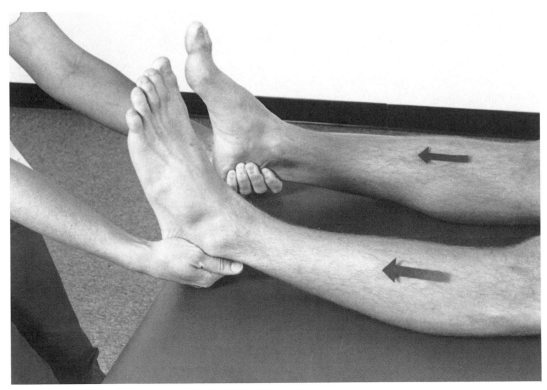

Figure 64: Hand position for the bilateral leg pull, with the patient supine.

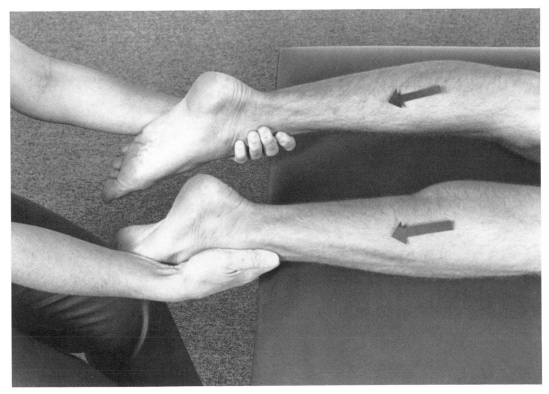

Figure 65: Hand position for the bilateral leg pull, with the patient prone.

The Bilateral Arm and Leg Pull:
Two-or Three-Person Stretch

Two people can perform simultaneous arm and leg pulls as described earlier (Figs. 66-69). Each must counterbalance the other's pull to avoid dragging the patient in either direction. Each person must apply traction firmly, wait for the release, and take up the slack again. If this traction is applied in a timid fashion, no true stretching will occur. If a third person is available while traction is applied to the patient's arms and legs, the third person performs a longitudinal stretch, focusing on the target musculature (Figs. 70-71). This maneuver will often achieve a degree of relaxation unachievable with any other methods, including mechanical traction.

Once the straight line stretch is completed, further stretch can be achieved by using the patient's arm and leg on the same side to release unilateral tightness (see the following), while stretching the opposite arm and leg in a diagonal pattern also releases the oblique muscles of the abdomen (see below).

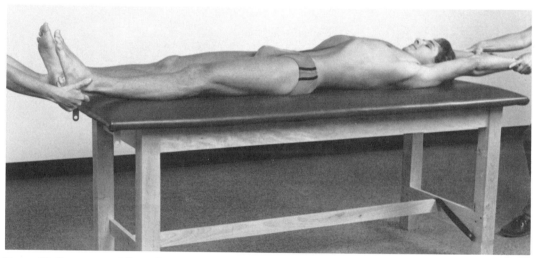

Figure 66: Two-person bilateral arm and leg pull, with the patient supine.

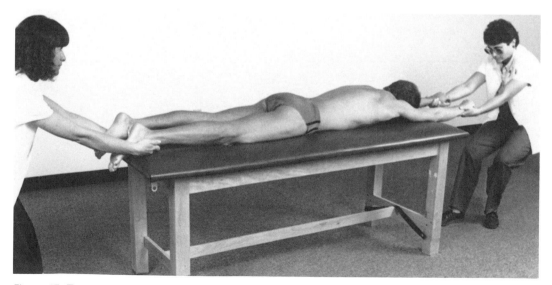

Figure 67: Two-person bilateral arm and leg pull, with the patient prone.

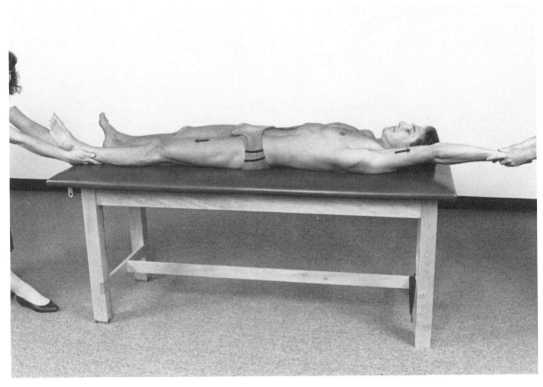

Figure 68: Two-person ipsilateral arm and leg pull, with the patient supine.

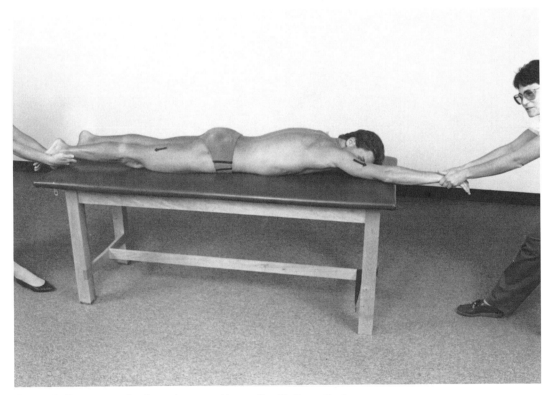

Figure 69: Two-person ipsilateral arm and leg pull, with the patient prone.

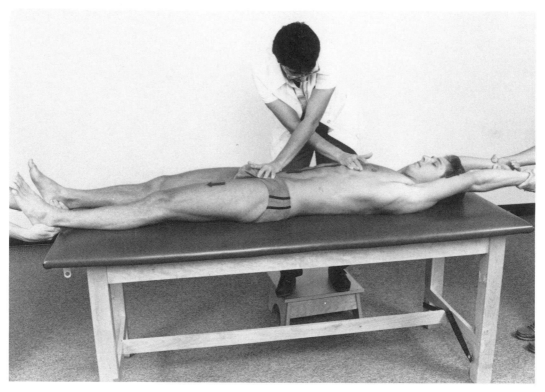

Figure 70: Three-person bilateral arm and leg pull, with longitudinal stretching of the abdominal muscles.

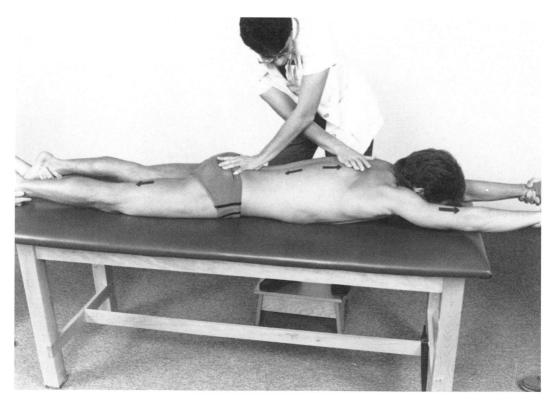

Figure 71: Three-person bilateral arm and leg pull, with longitudinal stretching of the erector spinae muscle.

The Bilateral Arm and Leg Pull: The Ipsilateral Stretch

Using the arm and leg on the same side of the body is a very effective means of stretching all muscles which do not easily lend themselves to stretching in any other fashion, including the latissimus dorsi, the quadratus lumborum, and the intercostal muscles. It is possible to take up the slack in these muscles more effectively than can be done when attempting to stretch the muscles directly. While the stretch can be done as a two-person technique, it is even more efficient using three people. The third person can do direct stretching while the other two people are engaged with the arm and leg pull (Figs. 72-74).

After instructing the patient to "lie heavily" on the table and not move the hips, take both of his arms and legs and stretch into a concave position (Figs. 75-76). Further stretch the restricted side through a full range of motion, reproducing the motion of lateral trunk flexion (Figs. 77-78).

The person in the middle with hands directly on the targeted muscle group should act as captain in this case. The stretch can be performed with the patient prone, supine, or side-lying. Multiple variations of the side-lying can be used, with the patient propped over a roll, several pillows, or allowed to lie directly on his side (Figs. 79-80).

The person in the middle should stretch the targeted muscle and then direct the two assistants to begin tractioning the arm and leg to take up the remaining slack in the muscle. Interestingly, the additional slack will not be detected until the arm and leg pull make it obvious, which is what makes it so difficult to stretch these muscles by oneself. Once again, the line of pull should be directed by the captain, depending upon the specific areas of tightness palpated and the feedback received from the patient's body.

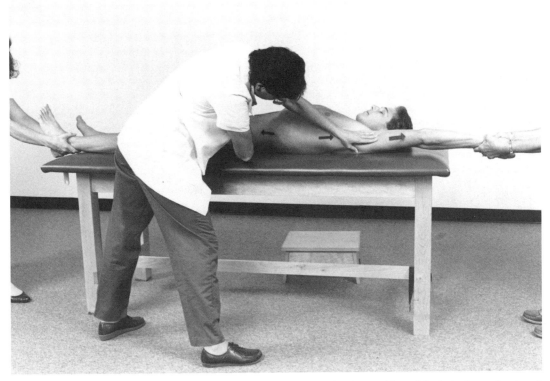

Figure 72: Three-person ipsilateral arm and leg pull, with longitudinal stretching of the latissimus dorsi and quadratus lumborum.

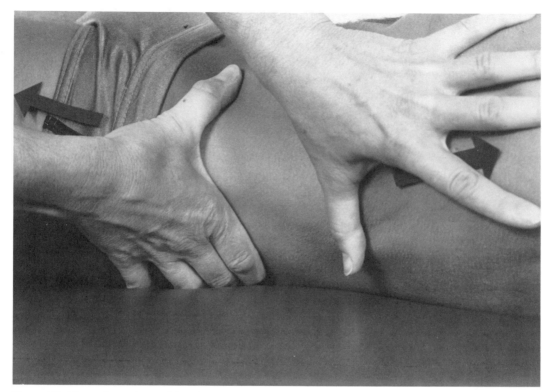

Figure 73: Close view of stretching the quadratus lumborum. Direct stretching of the lateral trunk musculature can focus on and stretch large or small muscle groups with equal ease.

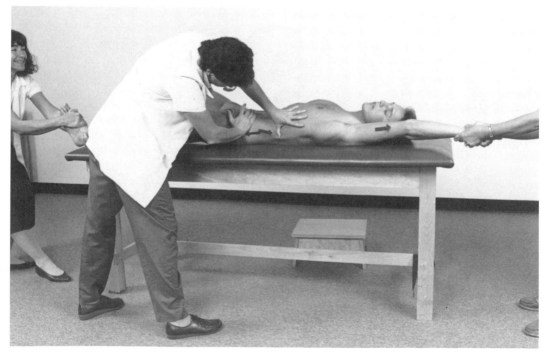

Figure 74: Three-person ipsilateral arm and leg pull, with longitudinal stretching of the quadratus lumborum muscle.

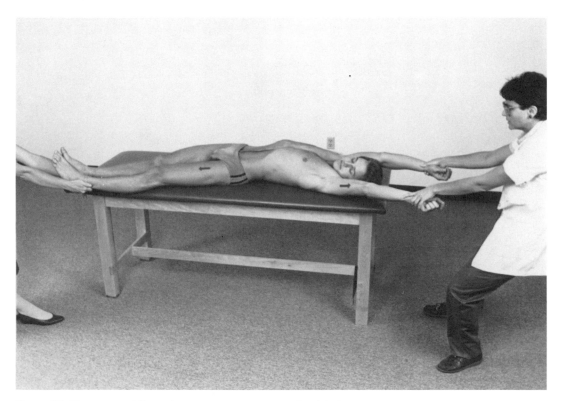

Figure 75: Two-person bilateral concave arm and leg pull, with the patient supine.

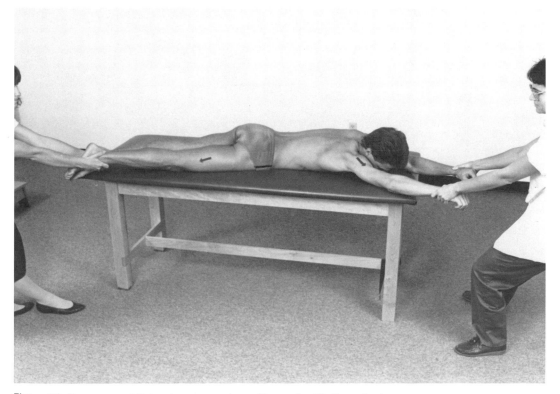

Figure 76: Two-person bilateral concave arm and leg pull, with the patient prone.

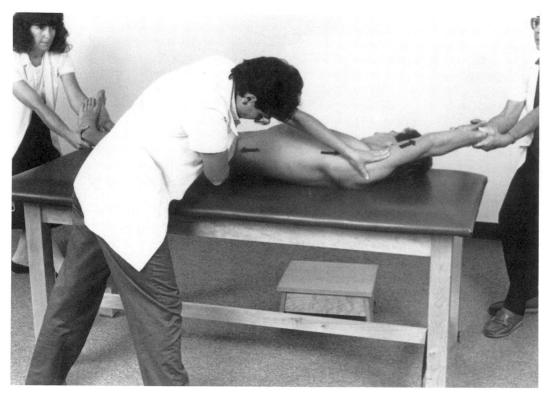

Figure 77: Three-person bilateral concave arm and leg pull, with longitudinal stretching of the latissimus dorsi. For this particular muscle, both the prone and supine positions allow almost the same accessibility.

A. In this view, hand placement for the stretching of the latissimus is shown on the covex side.

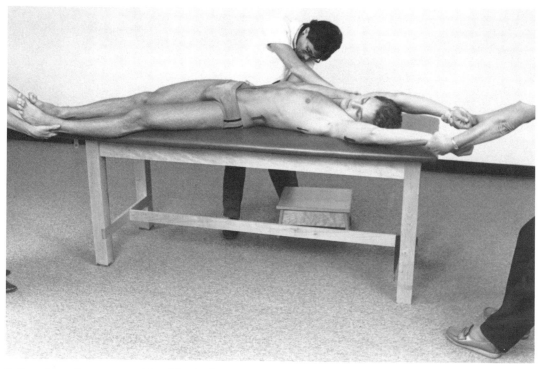

B. Seen from the concave side of the body.

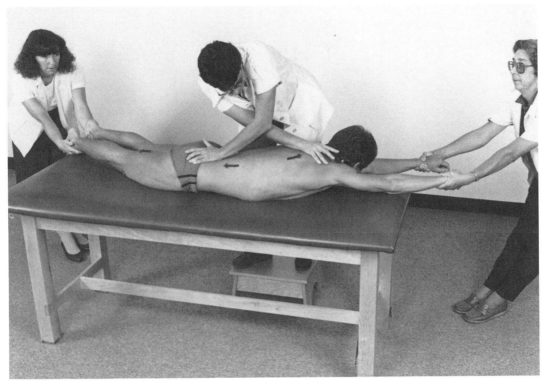

Figure 78: Three-person bilateral concave arm and leg pull, with longitudinal stretching of the erector spinae muscle with the patient prone.

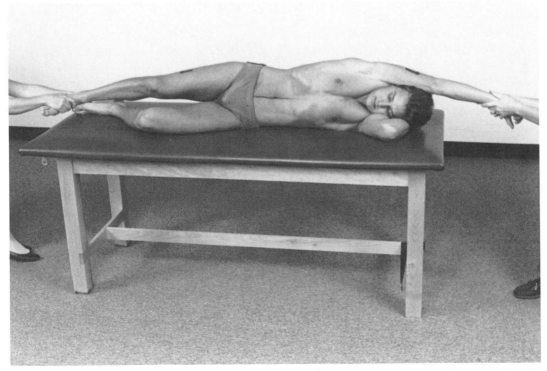

Figure 79: Two-person side-lying arm and leg pull. For an added stretch, a bolster can be placed directly under the target muscle.

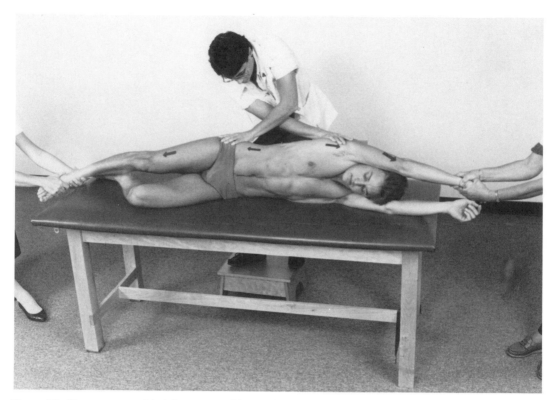

Figure 80: Three-person side-lying arm and leg pull, with longitudinal stretching of the latissimus dorsi muscles.

The Bilateral Arm and Leg Pull: The Contralateral Stretch

Using two or three people, a contralateral stretch is very effective in removing restrictions that cross the midline of the body. Your patient can be either prone or supine for this stretch. Depending upon the position, different muscle groups are emphasized. A prone position stretches the iliopsoas, the lower trapezius, and the serratus anterior. A supine position stretches the obliques, the pectorals and, to a lesser extent, the iliopsoas and the intercostals.

Visualize the line of stretch going from one arm to the contralateral leg, running though both obliques. Position yourself accordingly, with the person at the head acting as captain and directing the person at the leg (Figs. 81-82).

A restriction can encompass all fibers in a muscle or a subset of them. If the only restrictions present include all muscle fibers in every muscle being stretched, the arm and leg will be perfectly lined up and the releases will occur in a smooth sequential manner. If some restrictions do not include all the fibers of a muscle, then it will be necessary to change the angle of the arm, leg, or both in order to release them completely. Releases will then occur in a somewhat jerky fashion until all the restrictions are removed. At that point, line up the arm and leg as previously described and do a final maximal stretching of all muscles.

When using three people, the person in the middle should have his hands on the oblique muscles and will be the captain directing the other two team members (Figs. 83-84).

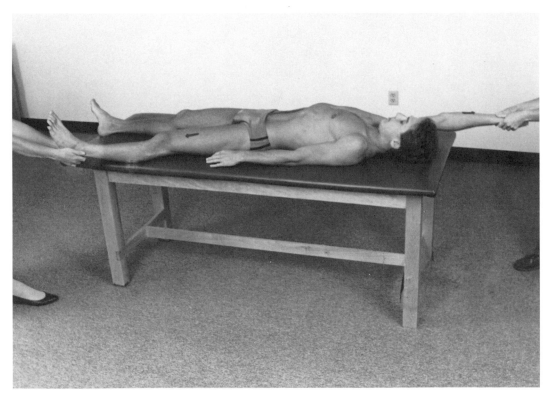

Figure 81: Two-person diagonal arm and leg pull, with the patient supine.

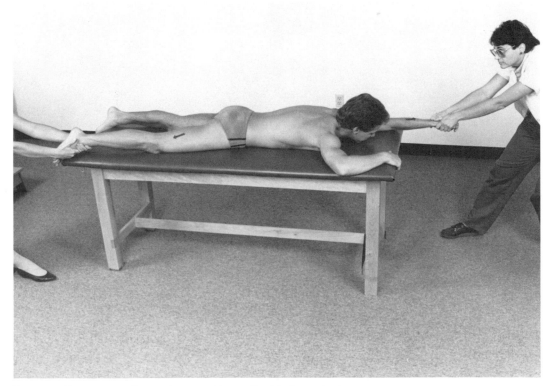

Figure 82: Two-person diagonal arm and leg pull, with the patient prone.

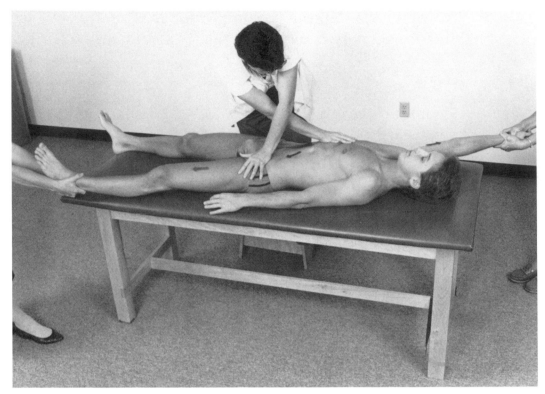

Figure 83: Three-person diagonal arm and leg pull, with longitudinal stretching of the oblique muscles.

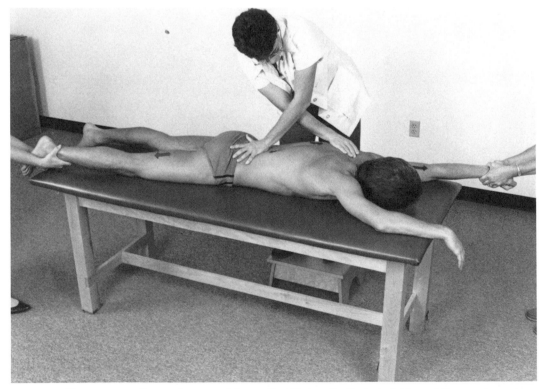

Figure 84: Three-person diagonal arm and leg pull, with longitudinal stretching of the erector spinae muscles.

Two-or Three-Person Technique for Stretching the Shoulder Portion of the Upper Trapezius Muscle

Often, it is very helpful to have an assistant placing traction on the arm while you are directing your attention to the shoulder portion of the upper trapezius, as described earlier. With a little practice, you will be able to direct your assistant to position the arm in the most efficient manner to facilitate releasing tension in the upper trapezius muscle and in the entire upper quarter as well. The person who is at the patient's head always acts as the captain of the team, directing other team members as to which direction and how much force to apply.

Once again, take your position at your patient's head. Place your hands on the upper trapezius, stretching laterally and slightly downward. As your assistant applies gentle traction, you will be able to direct the proper line of pull through the proprioceptive feedback you receive from your patient's body (Fig. 85). Direct your assistant to take up the available slack and wait for the releases to occur.

When two people are assisting, both arms should be pulled on a straight line with the muscle fibers, and you should apply lateral and downward pressure on both shoulders (Fig. 86). This results in symmetrical stretching of both of the upper trapezii muscles. If asymmetrical tightness is detected, you can then place both hands on that portion of the muscle which is restricted while your assistants continue to apply traction.

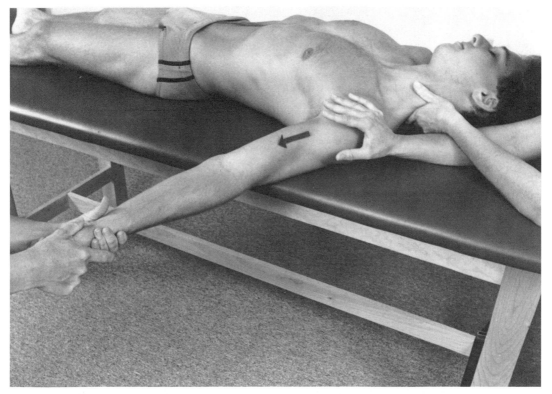

Figure 85: Two-person technique for stretching the shoulder portion of the upper trapezii muscles.

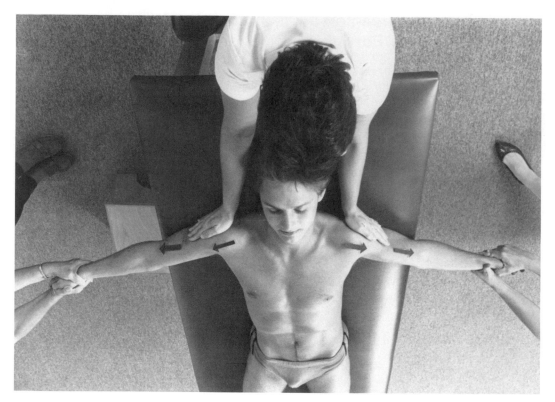

Figure 86: Three-person technique for stretching the shoulder portion of the upper trapezii muscles.

Stretching the Middle Trapezii Muscles

The middle trapezii muscles are often ignored in terms of stretching. When performing a bilateral arm pull, it is very easy to stretch this muscle as its fibers are horizontal and are very superficial and accessible to myofascial stretching. For the most efficient stretching of the middle trapezii, two assistants are needed to maintain traction on both arms. However, you can also stretch the middle trapezii muscles without assistants.

Once again, place your hands on the distal attachments of the muscle, stretch to take up the slack and wait until the release occurs (Fig. 87). If you have assistants, they should stretch the arms to take up any available slack there as well (Fig. 88). When focusing attention on the middle trapezii muscles, the arms should be perpendicular to the body and there should be very little tendency for the arms to move. However, as soon as the restrictions in the middle trapezii muscles are released, other restrictions will be quickly revealed and the line of pull will then correspond to the uncovered restrictions.

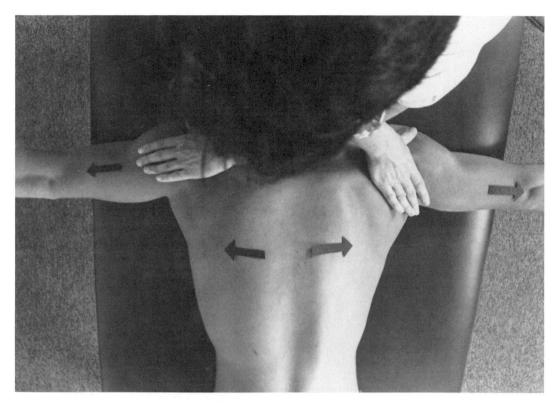

Figure 87: Stretching of the middle trapezii muscles.

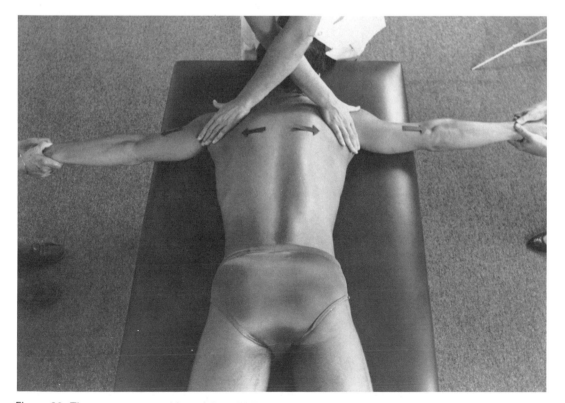

Figure 88: Three-person stretching of the middle trapezii muscles.

Stretching the Lower Trapezii Muscles

The lower trapezii are more often over-stretched by persistent tightness of the upper trapezii and the elevators of the scapulae. However, at times you might find it necessary to stretch the lower trapezii to help free scapular motion. As a one-person technique, the muscle is easily targeted and stretched in the usual manner (Fig. 89). Two people can stretch the lower trapezius in a more efficient manner by having one perform an arm pull along the direction of the fibers of the lower trapezius while the other uses the direct technique (Fig. 90). Obviously, for the arm pull to be effective, tightness above the level of the lower trapezius muscle must be cleared first.

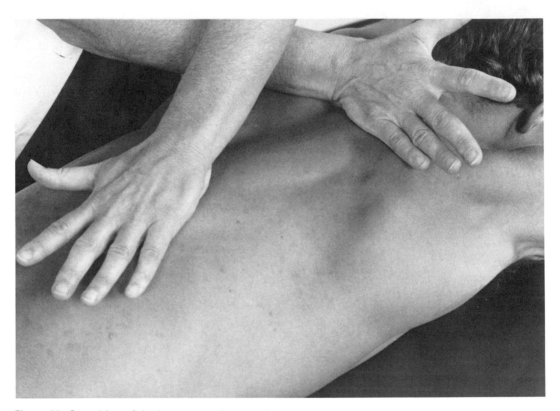

Figure 89: Stretching of the lower trapezius muscle.

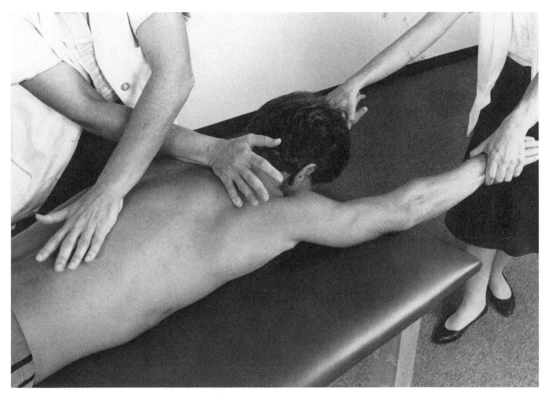

Figure 90: Two-person stretching of the lower trapezius muscle.

Two-or Three-Person Technique for Stretching the Pectoral Muscles

The pectoral muscles can be more effectively stretched when using a two-person technique. Have your assistant place traction on the arm in a line corresponding with the line of stretch of your hands (Figs. 91-92). Take up all the slack in the muscle, hold, wait for the release, and then stretch again. Direct your assistant to maintain the proper angle of the arm to the body as different fibers of the muscles are stretched. Continue this pattern until an end feel is reached. As the pectoralis major relaxes, your attention will be drawn to the pectoralis minor. The feedback you receive from your hands will direct your position for most efficient stretching. You may find that you no longer want the arm to be stretched while you are focusing your attention on the pectoralis minor. That decision will be based upon your growing sense of what feels right as you proceed with these techniques.

When the pectoral muscles are tight bilaterally, a three-person stretch may be used on the horizontal fibers (Fig. 93).

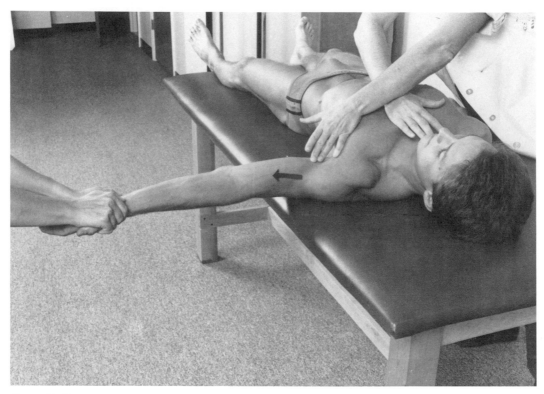

Figure 91: Two-person stretching of the horizontal fibers of the pectoral muscles.

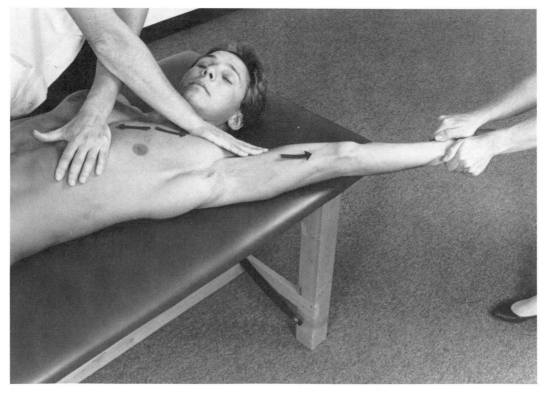

Figure 92: Two-person stretching of the lower fibers of the pectoral muscles.

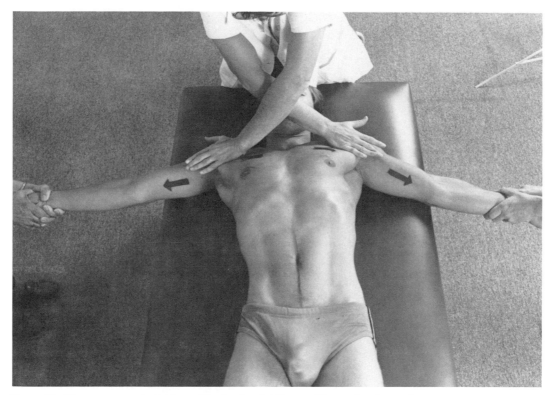

Figure 93: Three-person stretching of the horizontal fibers of the pectoral muscles.

Superficial Releases

Myofascial restrictions are sought when assessing skin mobility, starting with restrictions between the most superficial layers and working toward deeper layers. The movement of the skin over the underlying but superficial structures is checked first. Depending on the body part being tested, either the palm or the finger tips are used to detect restrictions. On broad body surfaces, the palm is firmly but lightly placed on the skin and then is pushed upward, downward, and from side to side to feel for free movement (Figs. 94-97).

Once superficial restrictions in skin mobility have been found, they are easily released by "J-stroking" across the restrictions. This technique does not rely on feedback from the patient, but is done with specific restrictions in mind. The J-stroking procedure is similar to connective tissue massage, with definite lines of stroking to be followed;[13] however, it is performed only in an area identified in the assessment as being restricted and not throughout a generalized area, as would be done with connective tissue massage. Once these superficial restrictions are released, myofascial release can be performed with greater ease because the feedback is not muted by the superificial skin restrictions.

To perform a superficial release, firm but gentle contact is required. The skin is stretched to take up any slack (Fig. 98). With the second and third fingers held against each other for added strength and stability, the therapist firmly draws short Js on the patient's skin, progressively moving across the restricted area. After the area is treated completely once, the area is reassessed and treated again with J-strokes until no further restrictions are found. Transient hyperemia will be present following this treatment. In addition, the patient may complain of a burning or tearing sensation with these releases, which is the same response as to connective tissue massage.[13]

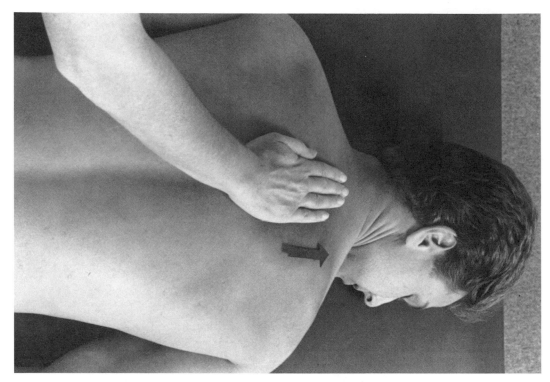

Figure 94: Testing for thoracic skin mobility. No restriction of movement is demonstrated in this series of illustrations.

A. Upward.

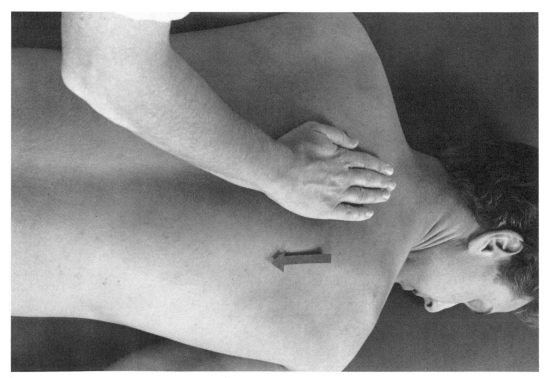

B. Downward.

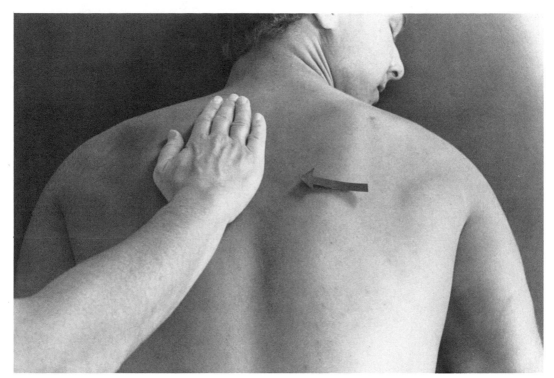

C. Left.

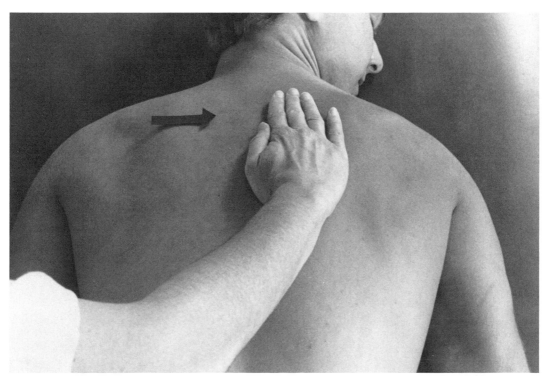

D. Right.

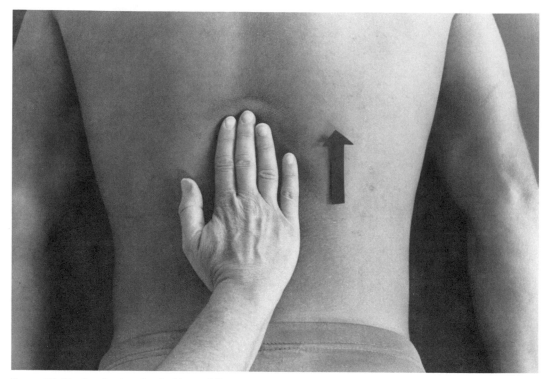

Figure 95: Testing for low back skin mobility.

A. Upward mobility is restricted. Note the bunching of the skin in front of the therapist's fingers.

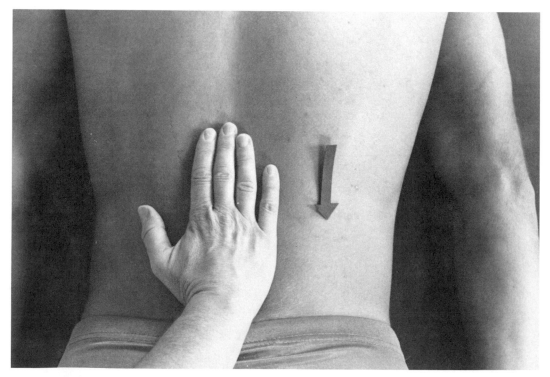

B. Downward.

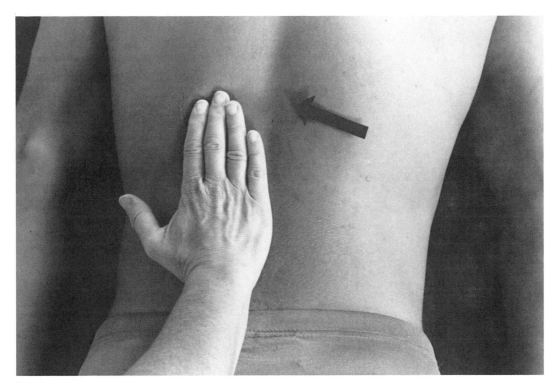

C. Left.

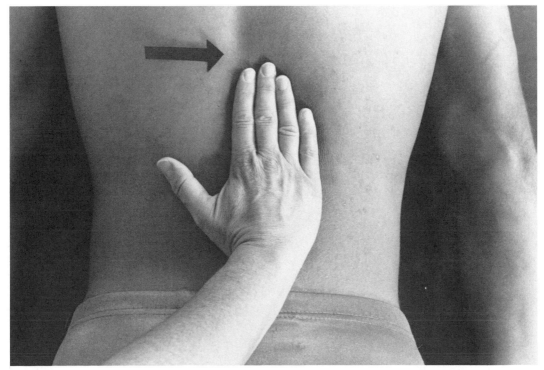

D. Right.

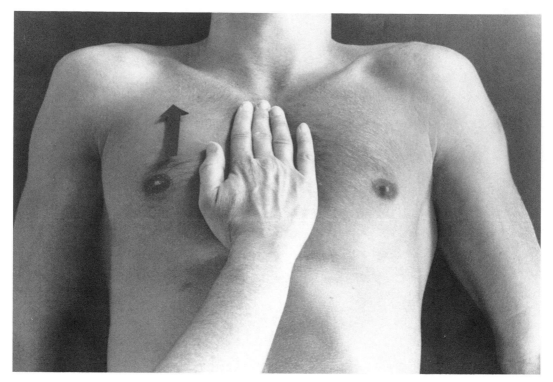

Figure 96: Testing for anterior chest wall skin mobility. No restrictions are demonstrated.

A. Upward.

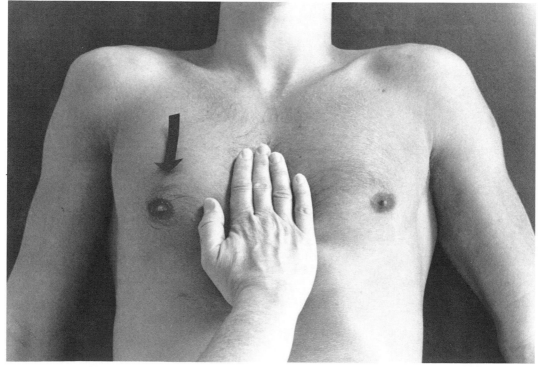

B. Downward.

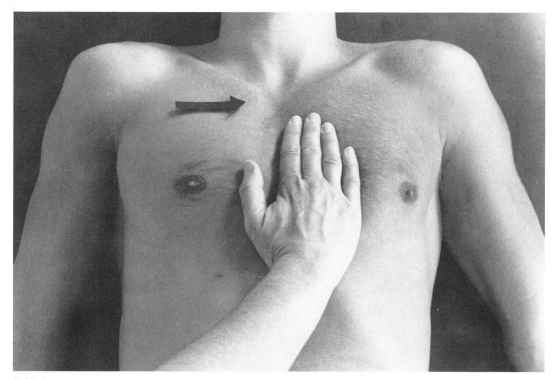

C. Right.

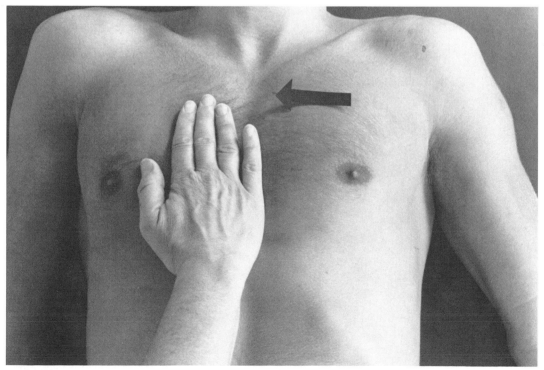

D. Left.

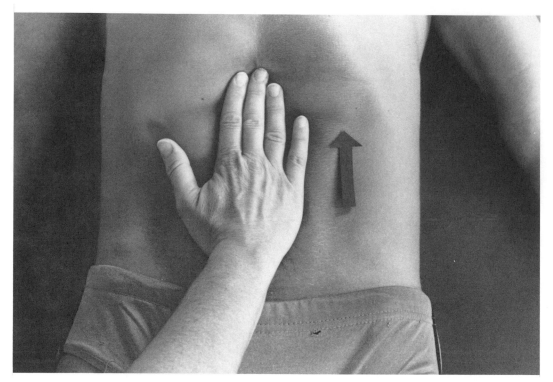

Figure 97: Testing for abdominal skin mobility.

A. Upward.

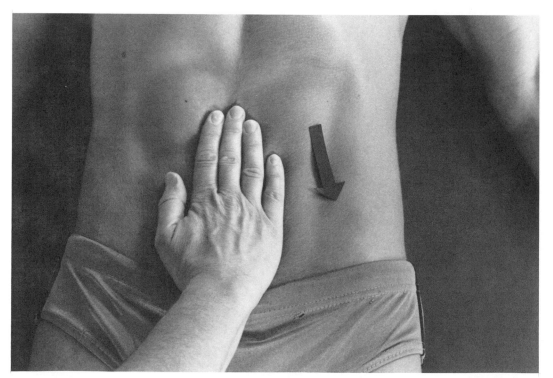

B. Downward.

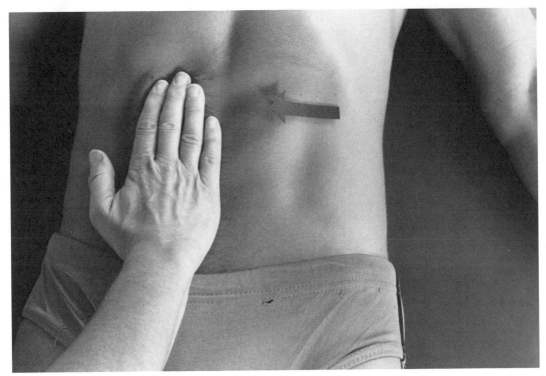

C. Left. Note the restriction of movement and the bunching of the skin by the therapist's hand.

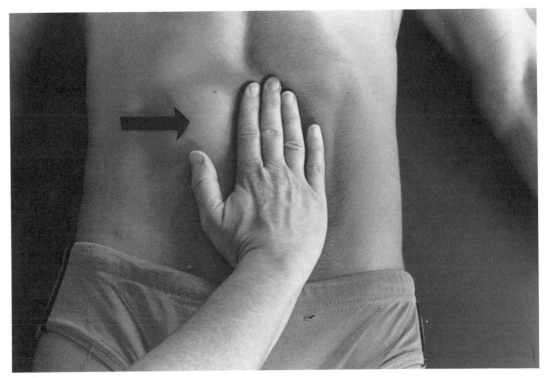

D. Right.

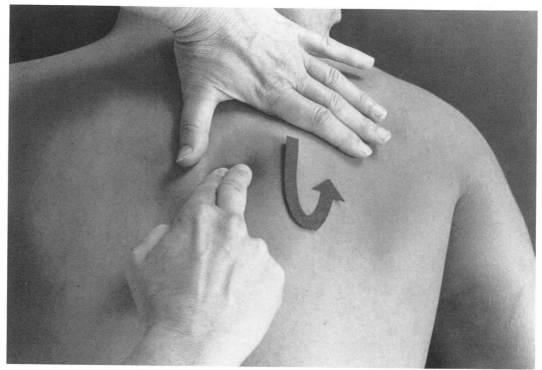

Figure 98: Hand placement for J-stroking. The upper hand must stretch and stabilize the skin above the area of restriction to eliminate extraneous movement which would prevent stretching of the restrictions.

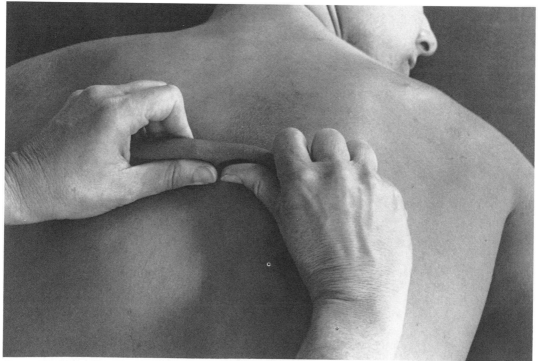

Figure 99: Skin rolling for the release of superficial restrictions.

Another method of releasing superficial restrictions is "skin rolling." In an area with no or minimal restrictions, the skin is rolled between the thumb and figures of the therapist. Gradually, the therapist rolls into the area of restriction. As restrictions are felt, slightly greater force is used to lift and pull the skin upward, forward, and backward, until all restrictions are released (Fig. 99). This same technique can be used to release scar tissue when enough area is available in which to work, such as in the abdominal or thoracic regions.

Trigger Points

Active myofascial trigger points are discrete, reproducible foci of hypersensitivity. When palpated, trigger points result in localized sharp, radiating, and referred pain.[14-27] This pain rarely, if ever, follows dermatomal or peripheral nerve distribution patterns.[25,28] Myofascial trigger point pain patterns are well documented.[14,18,22,23,25,29-46,64]

Active myofascial trigger points are perceived by the patient as being painful without stimulation. An active myofascial trigger point is always sensitive, restricts motion,[23,25,47-50] causes muscle weakness,[23,45] elicits protective muscle spasm with an adequate stimulus, and often produces predictable autonomic responses. These autonomic responses can include vasoconstriction, vasodilation, hypersecretion, global hypersensitivity, and pain either locally or distally with adequate stimulation.[14,19,23,25,45,51-55] In addition, they are areas of lowered skin resistance[54] and sometimes are associated with fibrositic nodules.[56-58] They may elicit the "jump sign" with palpation.[18,23,59]

The active myofascial trigger point can cause secondary trigger points in agonistic and antagonistic muscles that develop in response to overload, as those muscles try to compensate for or assist the injured muscle (splinting). Satellite trigger points can develop within the reference zone of the original active trigger point.[25] Latent trigger points are painful only with palpation[23,25,60] and may elicit the same sensory, autonomic, and motor phenomena with an adequate stimulus.

As hyperexcitable foci, myofascial trigger points respond to increasingly smaller stimuli over time.[14,23,25,61] Thus, patients who increasingly complain of pain are reporting a real phenomenon are not simply becoming chronic complainers.

Myofascial trigger points often are found in a taut band of skeletal muscle or fascia.[19,22,23,25,51,58,62] Other trigger points can also be found in scar tissue,[63] tendons, ligaments, skin, fat pads, joint capsules, and the periosteum. Trigger points which are not myofascial in origin do not cause the referred pain patterns or other referred problems, but rather function as local irritants. These trigger points must also be released to allow maximum relaxation of all restricted tissues and eradication of the localized pain.

Myofascial trigger points can cause or mimic many different problems. These problems defy diagnosis since they do not respond positively to the standard diagnostic tests or treatment for that problem. However, elimination of the myofascial trigger point will also completely eliminate the problem. Some of these problems are listed in Table 1.

The complaints listed in Table I are not contraindications to myofascial stretching but, rather, they are the indications for it. For example, the patient with angina-like pain and no known underlying cardiac cause should be treated with myofascial stretching and trigger point releases. Often, this patient will be found to have extreme tightness in the chest wall. The pain that mimics angina will disappear with successful myofascial stretching and trigger point elimination. Before embarking upon myofascial treatment, the therapist must be sure, however, that the patient's attending physician has thoroughly investigated all complaints and has found no other medical explanation for them.

Successfully treated medical problems may leave myofascial tightness that also responds quite effectively to myofascial stretching. Trigger points within mature scar tissue and the scar itself need to be released in order to allow free myofascial movement and to eliminate restrictions caused by adhesions. Although the sensation is usually quite painful and often perceived as knife-like and tearing, no reopening of the wound occurs. The release of restriction often dramatically gives back movement the patient was unaware of losing. Problems quite distal to, and seemingly unrelated to, a scar can be solved in this manner.

There is a reflex relationship between muscles which are under tension due to trigger points in one

Table 1
Problems Caused by Trigger Points

Symptom	Reference	Symptom	Reference
appendicitis	23, 38	muscle spasm	25
arthritic knee pain	23	occipital neuralgia	23, 25, 67, 72, 73
arthritic hip pain	23	otitis	23, 25
chest pain in typical anginal patterns	17, 23, 25, 35, 64, 65, 66	sciatica	23, 30, 37, 41, 99
		subdeltoid bursitis	20, 23, 25, 74
dysmenorrhea	23	tension headache	18, 23, 25, 64, 67, 75
epicondylitis	23, 25, 49	thoracic inlet syndrome	18, 23, 25, 37, 64, 67
facial neuralgia, atypical	23, 25, 44, 67, 68	tinnitus	46
fibromyositis	17	torticollis, acute	23, 25, 76
heel spur	23, 41, 49	tochanteric bursitis	23, 41
hiccups	69	vertigo	77
inguinal pain	70	vomiting, uncontrollable	25
jaw/TMJ pain	34, 47, 60, 67, 71		

of them. Thus, release of a trigger point in one muscle may, through reflex inhibition, also relax other muscles which are exhibiting increased tension. For example, relaxation of the gluteus maximus may eliminate pain and tenderness referred to the coccyx or the levator ani. Release of the suboccipital muscles may relax the sternocleidomastoid, and vice versa, while release of the thoracolumbar erector spinae muscles may relax the iliopsoas. The sternocleidomastoid and the scalene muscles reciprocally affect the pectoral muscles.[49,78]

Latent and active myofascial trigger points prevent maximal relaxation of the myofascial unit and, therefore, must be released in conjunction with myofascial stretching before a true end point is achieved. The therapist can be deceived into thinking maximal elongation has occurred when it has not, if trigger points are not located and released. The myofascial unit will return to its pre-treatment length within minutes, hours, or several days if all of the trigger points within it are not released. Therefore, even if the patient does not complain of point tenderness, less than optimal relaxation and stretching of the myofascial unit suggests that untreated or incompletely treated trigger points are present.

When performing myofascial stretching on a specific myofascial unit, the therapist initially needs to be concerned only with trigger points in that specific unit. If the stretch does not hold, the patient should be reassured that the solution to the problem will be found and that the setback is temporary. The therapist should also not get discouraged. He needs to realize that the puzzle is a bit more complicated than originally thought; is a challenge to be welcomed for what can be learned and applied to the treatment of other patients as well. The task for the therapist is to locate the primary trigger point that is influencing that myofascial unit.

The Manual Release of Trigger Points

Many different treatments have been used to eliminate trigger points with varying results. These included reflex inhibition following minimal or maximal isometric contraction,[49,67,70] ultrasound,[79] neuroprobe, electro-acuscope, dry needling,[45,80,81,82] anesthetic blocks,[14,30,36,37,46,70,83] intense cold,[14,38,44,45,67,77,84] TENS,[36] infra-red,[81] massage,[85] and ischemic pressure.[86] Often, a multi-faceted approach is needed along with myofascial stretching. The therapist should never become so limited and short-sighted as to rely on only one method of treatment to the exclusion of others. It is easy to forget some of the fine points of radiation patterns and treatment options. Therefore, I would suggest to even the most experienced and thorough therapist that periodic review is necessary.

The major factor in trigger point releases is determining which is the active, primary trigger point and which ones are secondary and satellite. Release of the primary trigger point not only eliminates that trigger point but also eliminates the secondary and satellite ones as well, along with associated sensory, motor, and autonomic phenomena.[25] The trigger points that are released visit after visit and return almost before the patient leaves the treatment room, are secondary or satellite points. Only when the primary ones are identified and released will lasting relief be gained by the patient.

The return of trigger points is a valid method for the therapist to use to determine which trigger points are not primary, but the puzzle of determining which ones are primary still remains. Because muscle relaxants temporarily eliminate secondary and satellite trigger points, thereby increasing pain from the primary trigger points because splinting is also temporarily eliminated,[25] a single dose of a muscle relaxant approximately two hours before assessment will allow the mapping of primary trigger points. However, this cannot be approached in a mechanical manner. The therapist must have confidence to allow patient feedback to guide his hands to the trigger points that need treatment.

It is always necessary to begin treating the most recent injury and the trigger points generated by it first and then to proceed backwards to old injuries and trigger points until lasting relief is obtained by the patient. This process will, of necessity, be spread over a number of treatments which is determined by the severity and the age of the injuries. In general, the older the injury, the more secondary and satellite trigger points will be generated, the more global the pain pattern will be, and the longer the treatment will take.

The initial goal of treatment then is to localize the pain pattern and more sharply define the location of the trigger points causing or existing within the pain pattern. As this puzzle is unraveled, the patient will begin to feel better and will be able to assist more actively in the localization and elimination of the trigger points that are the primary pain generators.

The therapist who is adept at myofascial release will be directed to these trigger points by feedback from the patient's body. The palpating fingers are drawn to the trigger point by the altered tissue tension. This altered tissue tension acts like a magnet which holds the therapist's attention until the trigger point has been neutralized and is no longer a pain focus.

Melzack found that 71% of acupuncture points used to treat pain corresponded with myofascial trigger points.[36] Therefore, an acupuncture chart can teach the beginner where to start looking for trigger points. The best reference to assist the therapist in locating trigger points is *Myofascial Pain and Dysfunction: The Trigger Point Manual* by Travell and Simons.[25] This text not only locates the primary trigger points but also shows the radiation patterns generated by the trigger points.

The trigger points can be layered on top of one another and must be released sequentially in a straight downward pressure. Alternatively, these trigger points can be proximal to each other and, as each one is released, the therapist's fingers float from layer to layer, releasing the trigger points as the hand is drawn successively to them.

Trigger points are released manually by applying carefully graded and gradually increasing pressure using a finger (Fig. 100), several fingers (Fig. 101), knuckles (Fig. 102), or an elbow (Fig. 103). The variations are limited only by the therapist's ingenuity and coordination. On occasion, more than one point will need to be released at the same time to break up a feedback pattern which perpetuates the trigger points.

When a trigger point is first located with gentle pressure, the patient will indicate either verbally or nonverbally that the location is correct. The therapist then applies slightly greater pressure, noting the radiation of the pain pattern, if any, and the location of any other trigger points in this referral zone. Next, the pressure is gradually increased to intensify the pain sensation at the trigger point being readied for a release. This intensification focuses the patient's attention on the trigger point and eliminates awareness of the reference zone.

Throughout, patient feedback directs treatment. The therapist works in concert and rhythm with the patient's body, increasing pressure as needed and easing back as needed. As the layers of the trigger point release, the therapist's hand is pulled more deeply into the offending tissues. At the point of final and total release of the trigger point, an emotional release may also occur. With or without the

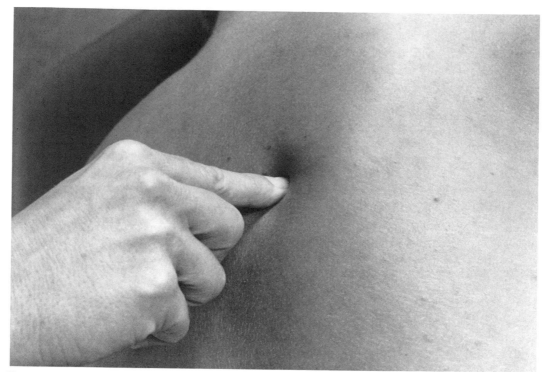

Figure 100: One-finger ischemic pressure on an active myofascial trigger point.

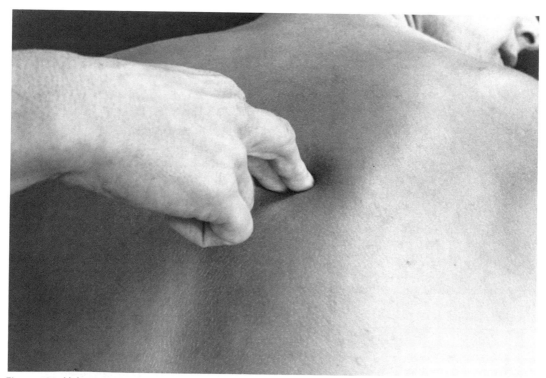

Figure 101: Using several fingers for ischemic pressure on an active myofascial trigger point.

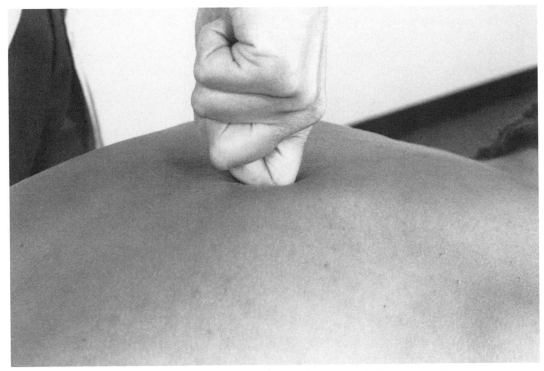

Figure 102: Using a knuckle for ischemic pressure on an active myofascial trigger point.

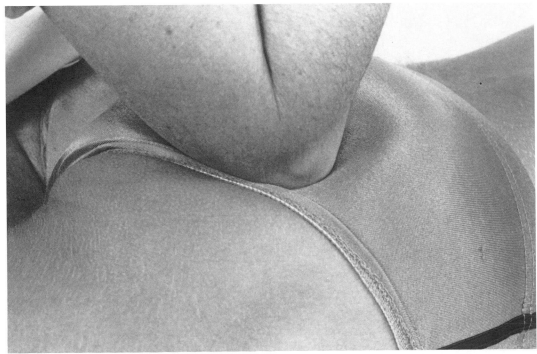

Figure 103: Using the elbow for ischemic pressure on an active myofascial trigger point on a deeper muscle such as the piriformis.

emotional component, the altered tissue tension slowly disappears, releasing the therapist from its grip. However, another nearby point may claim immediate attention and start the cycle anew with little pause.

Prior to a trigger point release, tell your patient that the release will be painful, but time-limited, and encourage him to express the pain verbally or to let the tears flow. Do not take personally anything a patient says during a trigger point release which can be very abusive and negative as his pain increases and peaks. Your patients will recognize the need and efficacy of this treatment if all previous attempts at eliminating the trigger point(s) have had limited or no success. I have always told my patients that I will stop if they want want me to, but none has ever done so. The sensation is one of a "good hurt," necessary, but painful. The whole key to successful trigger point releasing lies in the therapist being able to allow patient feedback to direct treatment, being empathetic and caring, and conveying this through his touch.

Release of the trigger points must be considered a deep and painful technique. Although trigger point releases are patient guided, most patients will have little active participation in the release. When using deep pressure to release the trigger points, the patient must be given an "out" word and permission to stop the release if the pain becomes intolerable. The therapist should first explain to the patient that if he can allow the pain to increase and reach maximum intensity, the release will be more complete and will allow the greatest amount of relaxation of the myofascial tissues. Even so, for long-standing trigger points, two or even more sessions may be needed to eradicate fully the offending trigger points that are preventing full elongation of the myofascial unit.

Strumming

Strumming is a very painful deep release technique. Before beginning this technique, the therapist must give the patient an "out" word to use if the pain is more than the patient is willing or able to tolerate. I use strumming only when more gentle techniques do not help.

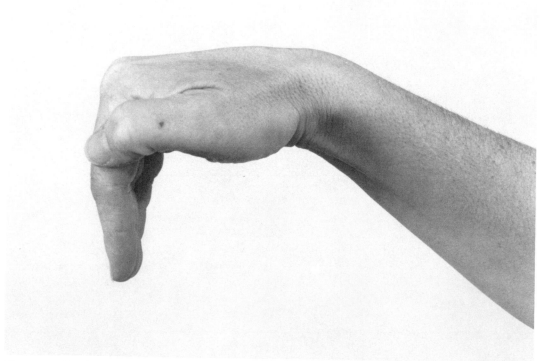

Figure 104: Hand position for strumming.

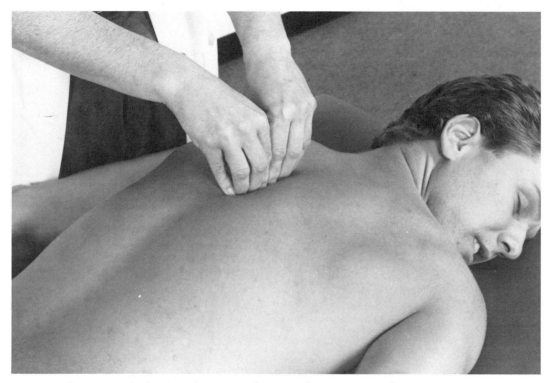

Figure 105: Strumming in the thoracic erector spinae muscles.

Strumming can be used around the knee to release the patella when abnormal tracking is present, along the erector spinae, to break up long-standing hypomobility of one or more vertebrae and at the adductor attachments to increase the available range of motion during a leg pull. Strumming is frequently used on the attachments along the ischial tuberosities and around the joints. As with J-stroking, strumming is similar to connective tissues massage,[13] but is used in a specific area and not as a general technique.

Strumming should be followed by interferential TENS and ice to decrease the tendency to swell and for its superficial analgesic properties. If the patient does not tolerate ice, use moist heat, interferential TENS, ultrasound, or any other modality that you prefer.

Strumming is usually performed with the fingers held in rigid extension (Figs. 104-105). Pressure is gradually applied to the restricted site by motion either perpendicular to or parallel to the muscle fibers. A back and forth scrubbing motion is then used to break loose the deep myofascial restrictions.

Alternately, you may cup your hand into a claw-like position (Fig. 106) and use a windshield wiper motion with deep pressure across and perpendicular to the muscle fibers.

Strumming is very tiring for the therapist's hands if it is performed for a long period of time. In this instance, "long" may be defined as thirty seconds to one minute or longer.

Strumming can also be performed using the elbows (Fig. 107) or knuckles (Fig. 108). In this instance, a long, deep stroking motion is used along the length of the myofascial unit. This type of strumming is used especially along the tensor fascia lata, the hamstrings, and the erector spinae muscles.

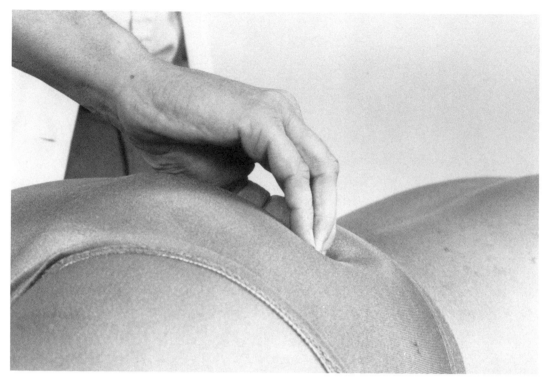

Figure 106: Claw-hand position for strumming larger muscle groups.

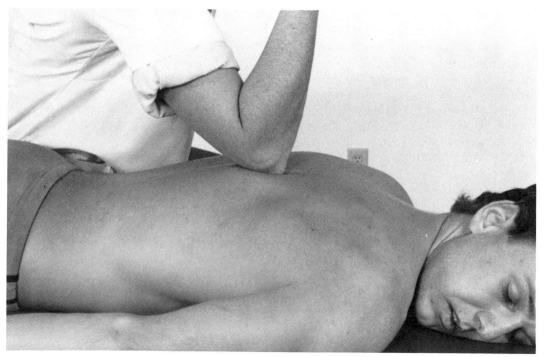

Figure 107: A. Long-stroking strumming using the elbow. Note the progression of stroke in pictures A through E.

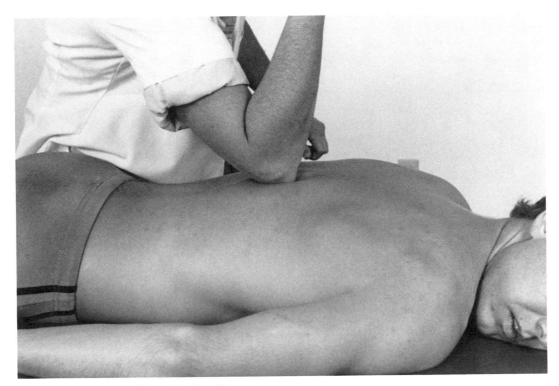

B. Long-stroking strumming using the elbow.

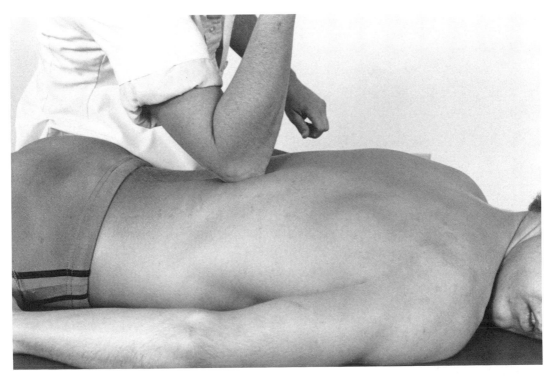

C. Long-stroking strumming using the elbow.

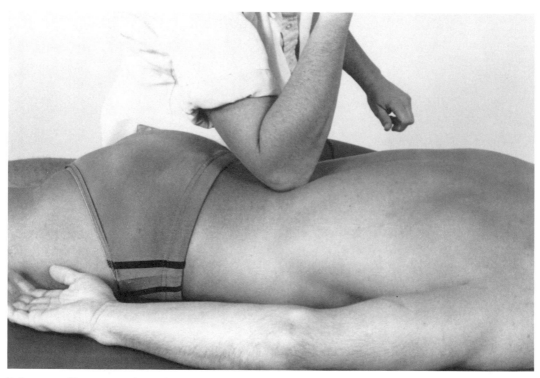

D. Long-stroking strumming using the elbow.

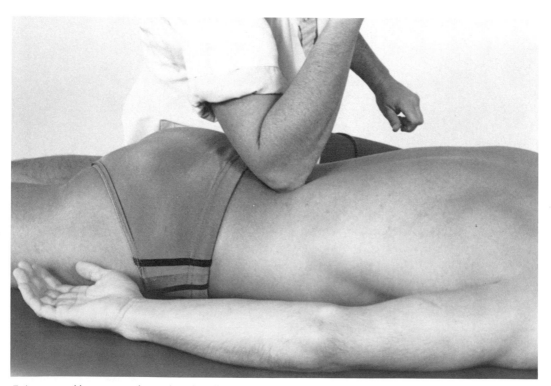

E. Long-stroking strumming using the elbow.

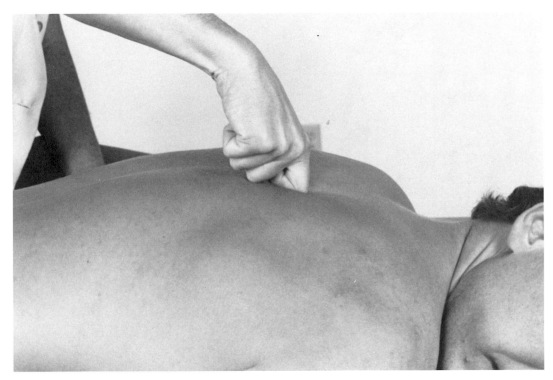

Figure 108: A. Long-stroking strumming using a knuckle. Note the progression of the stroke in pictures A through D.

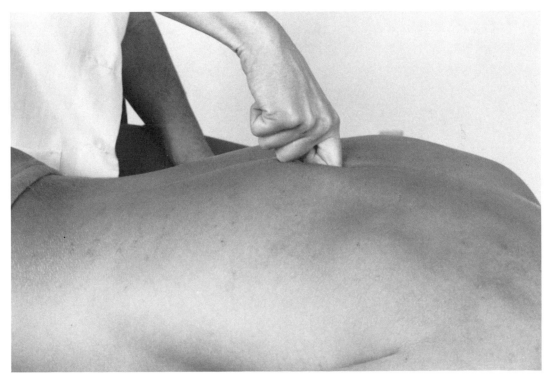

B. Long-stroking strumming using a knuckle.

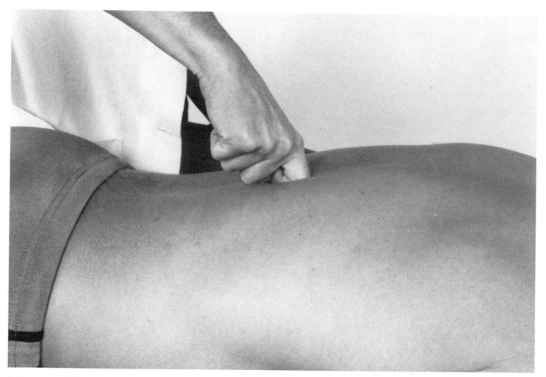

C. Long-stroking strumming using a knuckle.

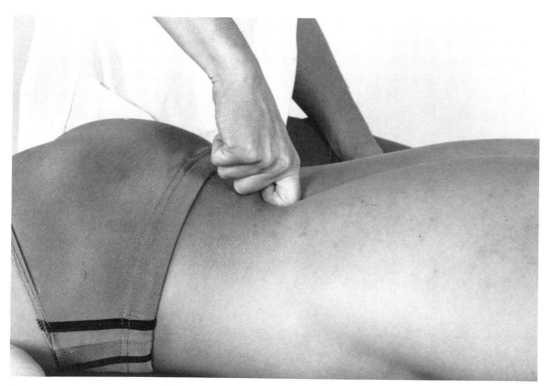

D. Long-stroking strumming using a knuckle.

Scar Release

Scars limit movement through adhesions. Scars can be moved in the same way as broad skin areas (Figs. 94-97) or by being gently pinched and lifted out from the body (Fig. 109).

Scar releases have been mentioned several different times in other sections (see trigger points and superficial releases). Release of scars must be considered a deep release technique no matter the method used, due to the intense pain the release causes. The age of the scar does not affect its potential for being released. Any healed scar can and should be released.

To release a scar, stroke slowly along the length of the scar while asking your patient to identify the most sensitive point in that scar. Once the most sensitive point is located, rotate your palpating finger in a clockwise direction, again asking your patient to identify the most sensitive point (Fig. 110). Now proceed with a trigger point release, gradually increasing your pressure as the superficial tissue relaxes, drawing your finger deeper into the restricted tissue.[63] Your patient will complain of increasing pain until the release occurs, at which point he may ask if you have released your pressure when, in fact, you have not.

Any scar may require more than one treatment session before the full available stretch is achieved and it is fully mobile. If the scar is still adherent to any degree following the first treatment, then at each subsequent visit, the release should be repeated until a final end feel is reached or the scar is fully mobile.

A deeply indented scar such as one from a healed abscess can be released in the same manner as a muscle is stretched. Place your hands on either side of the scar (Fig. 111). Stretch the skin between your hands by moving them away from each other until no further movement is possible. Hold until a release is felt and then stretch again. When no further stretch is possible in that direction, reposition your hands so you are stretching the scar at a right angle to your original line of stretch. Proceed as before. If the scar is not completely released, again move your hands 45 degrees away from your

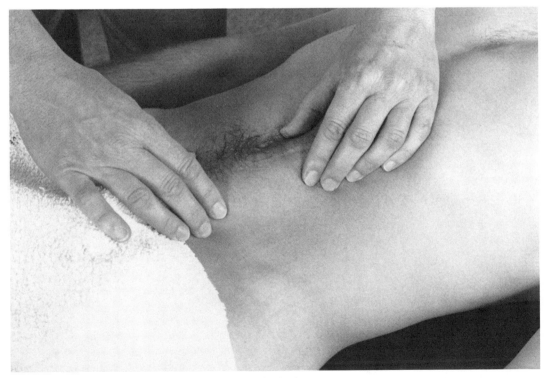

Figure 109: Scar release by lifting scar away from the body.

A. The scar is gathered in a pincer grip and lifted directly and slowly upward from the body, waiting as the soft tissues release, allowing greater distraction of the scar from the body.

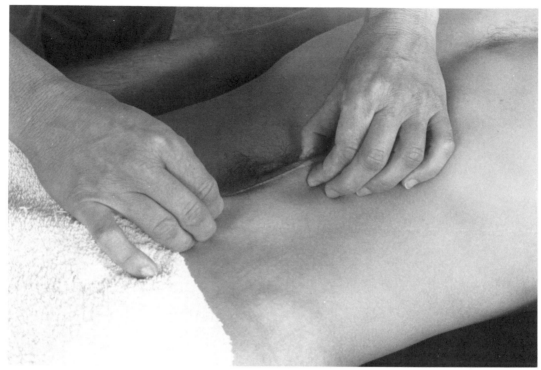

B. Once a full stretch away from the body is completed, the entire scar is moved to the left, again waiting for the soft tissues to release.

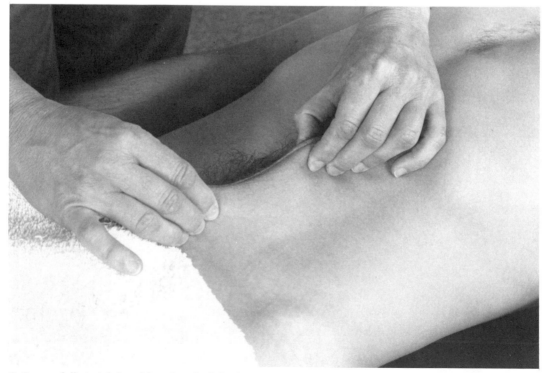

C. Once a full stretch is achieved to the left, the scar is gently and slowly pulled to the right, maintaining traction on the scar and waiting for the soft tissue releases.

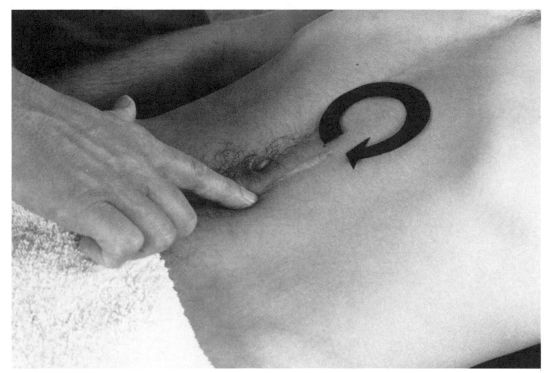

Figure 110: Finding the most sensitive part of the scar.

A. Run your finger down the entire length of the scar several times, asking your patient to tell you each time where the scar is the most sensitive.

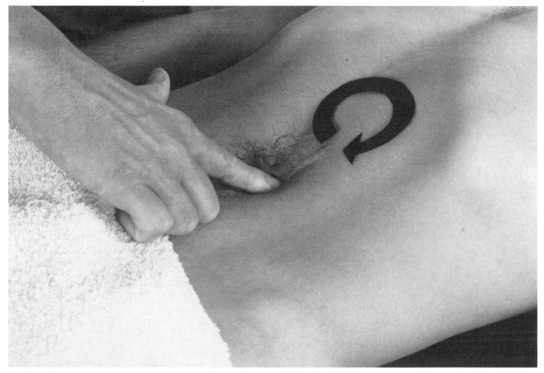

B. Once having located the most sensitive point, apply just enough pressure to keep your finger from slipping off that point.

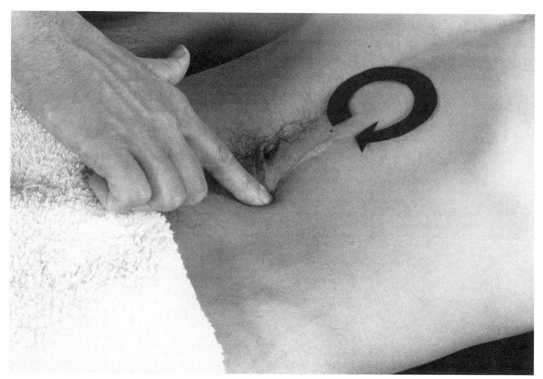

C. Keeping in contact with the original point, draw the skin around in a circle, again asking your patient to indicate where the scar is most sensitive.

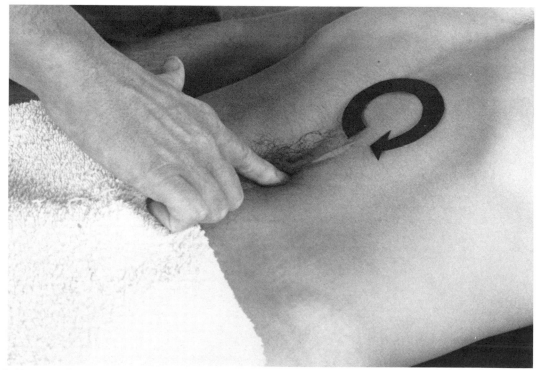

D. When the final determination of the most sensitive point on the scar is located, begin applying increasing pressure to that point, following the inherent tissue motion until a reduction in subjective pain is achieved.

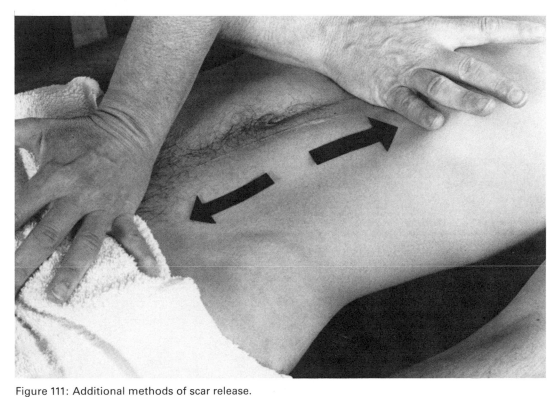

Figure 111: Additional methods of scar release.

A. Longitudinal stretching of a scar is approached the same way as stretching a long muscle group.

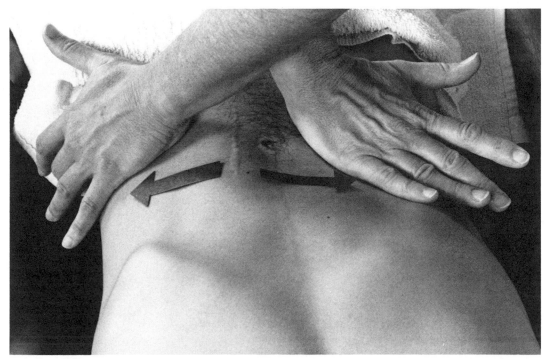

B. After achieving maximum stretch in the longitudinal direction, it is necessary to repeat the stretch at a 90 degree angle from the original stretch. This horizontal stretch of the scar will release additional restrictions still present even though the scar is fully mobile in the longitudinal direction.

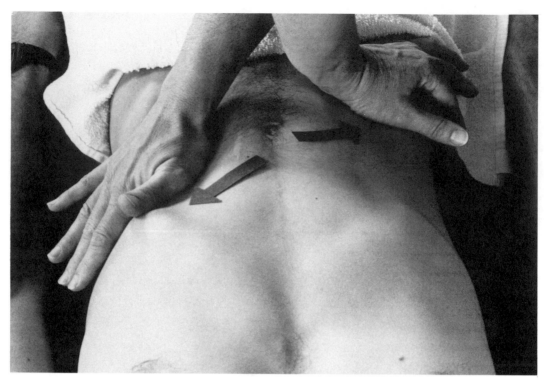

C. The final restrictions will be found with diagonal stretching of the scar at a 45 degree angle from the original stretch.

previous line of stretch and repeat the release procedure. You may need to repeat these releases during another treatment session(s) until the maximum available release is achieved. Even though an end feel is reached at the first treatment, the releases should be repeated if any amount of adherent scar remains.

Scars may also be released by using skin rolling, as described earlier (Fig. 99). This is also a good final technique to use to verify that all restrictions have been eliminated. Skin rolling is also used as an evaluation technique to determine if a scar is fully mobile or adherent when obvious restrictions are not present.

Balancing the Dural Tube

Balancing the dural tube is the connecting technique between myofascial release and craniosacral therapy. While it is an essential element in craniosacral therapy, balancing of the dural tube is not always needed when performing myofascial release. However, there are times when myofascial release cannot be accomplished in the usual manner and nothing seems to work. A restriction is sensed rather than felt; in spite of all the stretching you have done, something just does not feel right.

There are four instances when balancing of the dural tube is clearly indicated when performing myofascial release. First, the patient is symmetrical while lying on the table, but as soon as he gets up, all of the correction disappears. Second, the myofascial unit which you are trying to stretch remains unresponsive or responds in a minimal fashion. This most often will occur in long muscles such as the erector spinae or the abdominal muscles. Third, the correction disappears as soon as you release your hold. This is most likely to occur following a cranial base release, and it feels like a taut rubber band abruptly returning to its nonstretched length. Fourth, you perceive a feeling through your hands that something still needs to be released, but are unable to identify the specific structure. Balancing of the dural tube in these situations makes the difference between a successful treatment session and an unsuccessful one.

For example, I was working with a patient who had chronic neck and low back pain and who had active myofascial trigger points and myofascial restrictions in the abdomen. Manual trigger point releases were only partially successful, as was using the spray and stretch technique. My assistant and I tried a two-person longitudinal stretch and were unable to relax the abdominal muscles. They remained taut and unyielding until the dural tube was released. As soon as the dural tube was released, the abdominal muscles relaxed in a wave-like manner in a matter of seconds after the longitudinal stretch was begun again.

This technique is completely indirect. You cannot put your hands directly on the dural tube and your feedback is muted. Clinically, once you have perfected the technique, there will be no question that the technique works.

The full explanation of how and why balancing the dural tube works is still to be found. In fact, it is not at all clear whether the dural tube is actually being stretched or balanced by these techniques. Equally unclear is what restriction is being eliminated. Given this uncertainty, the following is an explanation of what Upledger believes is happening in the dural tube. Whether or not his explanation is correct, it is clear that the dural tube changes in concert with normal physiological movement.

Effects of Tension on the Dural Tube

Upledger considers the bones of the cranial vault as hard places within the dural membrane system. The cranial bones, the sacrum, and the coccyx are levers to be used in the evaluation and treatment of abnormal tension.[1] Upledger contends that abnormal tension in the dural membrane system is the most frequent and clinically significant cause of dysfunction. This abnormal tension is reflected histologically in the arrangement of fibers in the dural membranes, which align in the direction of tension.

Anatomy of the Dural Membrane System

The brain is soft and gelatinous, while the spinal cord is of a slightly firmer consistency. The meninges, skull, and vertebral column with its associated ligaments protect the central nervous system. These associated ligaments consist of the dura mater, which is the thick outer layer lined by the more delicate arachnoid and the thin pia mater. The pia mater adheres to the surfaces of the brain and spinal cord. In addition, the pia mater and the arachnoid line the subarachnoid space, which is filled with the cerebrospinal fluid.

The dura mater and the cerebrospinal fluid provide the main support and protection of the brain and the spinal cord. The cranial dura mater is attached to the periosteum lining the internal surfaces of the skull. This periosteum is continuous with the periosteum on the external surface of the skull at the margins of the foramen magnum and the smaller foramina for the nerves and blood vessels.[87]

The cranial dura mater is a dense, firm layer of collagenous connective tissue which is highly innervated and vascularized. The spinal dura mater is a tube which is pierced by the roots of the spinal nerves and which extends from the foramen magnum to the second sacral segment. The spinal dura mater is separated from the wall of the spinal canal by the epidural space which contains adipose tissue, the venous plexus, and cerebrospinal fluid. The spinal dura mater is also highly vascularized and innervated. For a detailed description of this innervation see Barr and Kiernan.[87] Suffice to say, the cranial dura mater and the spinal dura mater have a large sensory innervation so that distortions in the dura are rapidly transmitted throughout the central nervous system and, to a lesser extent, to the peripheral nervous system.

Normal Movement of the Dural Membrane System

Movements of the head and spinal column cause a physiologic change in shape of the hind brain and the cord.[88] This change in shape is due to the plastic adaptation of the nervous tissue as the spinal column changes length and shape with normal movement. The dura folds and unfolds in an accordion manner between the vertebrae, allowing free movement of the nervous tissue. If soft tissue restrictions or bony abnormalities prevent the normal movement of the dural tube, normal movement of the nervous tissue is also prevented. In contrast, a flexible dural tube can allow significant bony abnormalities to be present without nerve root impingement and can even accommodate a frankly ruptured disk without neurologic impingement (see below). Therefore, minimal neurologic changes can be present with significant bony abnormalities, and significant neurologic abnormalities can be present with minimal bony changes.

There is a significant difference in the mobility of the anterior and posterior surfaces of the cervical and lumbar dura. This is reflected in the different anatomical arrangements of the dura. The dorsal dura, an inelastic membrane, moves by unfolding of the accordion-like folds, while the ventral dura is attached to the posterior surfaces of the vertebral bodies and is held immobile by the nerve roots.[89-91]

When the head is rotated, the cervical canal narrows as the atlas, along with the dura mater, is rotated laterally. The lumen is made smaller by the folds of the dura in much the same way a camera lens is made smaller by the closing of the diaphragm.[88] Thus, if the dura is tight, even a minimal disk protrusion or bony abnormality will give rise to pain and dysfunction.[92]

In normal subjects, forward flexion of the head increases dural tension.[92] As the subject is urged to touch the chin to the chest to reach the end range of forward flexion, the dura is placed under greater tension. The dorsal portion of the dura between the occipital bone and the sacrum is 0.5 cm longer than the ventral portion.[88] Using cadavers, Brieg was able to show that the pia mater was stretched and ultimately transmitted the resulting tension to the lumbosacral nerve roots and to the sacral cone when the cervical spine was forward flexed with the trunk held erect.[90]

With hyperextension of the head, the entire dural tube is shortened, allowing the dura, spinal cord, and nerve roots to slacken.[90] The anterior surface of the dura relaxes and forms accordion-like folds at the level of the disks. This allows the anterior dura to protrude slightly into the spinal canal. At the same time, the lateral and posterior surfaces of the dura which lie between the vertebral arches fold and protrude into the spinal canal. Since the dura is attached to the arches by connective tissue, it does not move freely within the canal.[88] Thus, during forward flexion of the head, the cervical nerve roots are displaced upward in the neural foramina. This increases the angle between the nerve roots and the dura,[93] and potentially causes nerve root compression if the foramina is narrowed for any reason or if the dura is abnormally tight. The greatest potential for shortening and elongating of the dural tube lies in the posterior part of the cervical vertebral canal.

Lateral flexion of the head causes folding of the dura on the concavity and smoothing or stretching on the convexity. There is potential for nerve root compression on the convex side as the nerve root is displaced upward and on the concave side as the vertebrae approximate.

Axial folding of the dura is present in the atlanto-occipital junction, in the lower cervical region, and in the lower thoracic region with the erect posture. The axial dural folds deepen between the atlas and occiput with head rotation. The folds become slightly oblique with this rotation. The greater the amount of rotation, the further distally the effect is observed on the dura.[88]

In the lumbar region, lordosis and kyphosis produce similar movement of the dura. In maximum kyphosis, Brieg found that the posterior portion of the dural tube was elongated 2.2 mm,[88] while Charnley determined that the lumbar spine varied 5 mm between extreme flexion and extension.[91] If this movement is distributed over the whole length of the lumbar vertebrae, then each extradural root has to accommodate a very small amount of movement. Therefore, when a patient is asked to perform a pelvic tilt exercise, elongation and stretching of the posterior portion of the dural tube occurs. If the patient is then also asked to lift the head, touching chin to chest, the dural tube is placed on maximum stretch, transmitting tension from the sacrum to the occiput and from the occiput to the sacrum.

Pain as an Indicator of Dural Tube Restriction

Pain from the dura mater defies the rules of segmentation of the nervous system as well as anatomic limitations. Thus, a lesion in the cervical region can cause pain radiation from the mid-neck down to the scapulae, to the temple and forehead, and behind both eyes. This lesion in essence covers the distribution of twelve dermatomes.[94] The wide distribution of pain is due to the innervation of the dura mater by the sinuvertebral nerves along three separate routes. Only the ventral aspect of the dura is innervated.[95] For a detailed discussion of the pain structures within the neural canal, see Massey.[96] Irrespective of the area of the dura mater which is restricted, dural pain is provoked by coughing, and in this manner mimics a ruptured intervertebral disk.

Testing for Dural Tube Restriction

Individuals with low postural tone often assume a modified fetal position when upright. Maitland uses this position to test for dural tube restrictions.[12] In this case, it is called the Slump Test. Overpressure is placed on the spine once a fully rounded position is assumed. Stretching of the dural tube is increased by having the patient extend one knee and dorsiflexing the foot. Pain would indicate dural tube restrictions.[96]

Straight-leg raising tests dural mobility from the fourth lumbar vertebra downwards.[12,89,94] Dural tube restrictions are assumed to be present when neck flexion results in low back pain and when pain in the low back during straight-leg raising increases with neck flexion. Cyriax and Maitland advocate treating these restrictions with spinal manipulation, while Barnes and Upledger use the following dural tube releasing.

Releasing the Dural Tube: One-Person Technique

Ask your patient to lie on his side with his head slightly forward flexed and with hip and knees flexed into the fetal position. Use a pillow to maintain his head in neutral lateral flexion (Fig. 112). You should be sitting on a stool next to the plinth midway between your patient's head and buttocks. Place one hand on his occiput, cupping the occiput in your palm and allowing your fingers to extend lightly on the back of his head. Place your other hand on his sacrum so that the heel of your hand is at the top of the sacrum and your fingers extend downward over the body of the sacrum (Figs. 113-114).

Gently push the head upward and forward while pushing the sacrum downward and forward (Fig. 115). Hold until a release is felt and proceed as you would for any other release sequence or until spontaneous movement begins. If spontaneous movement begins, allow your hands to follow it as you

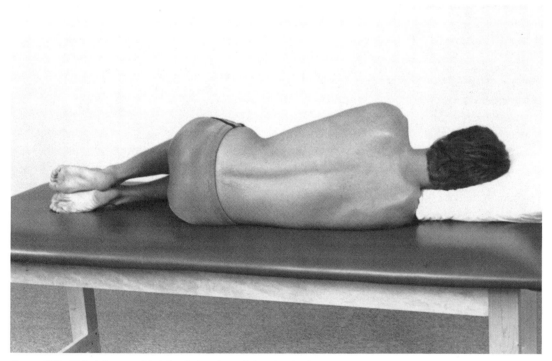

Figure 112: Side-lying position for balancing of the dural tube.

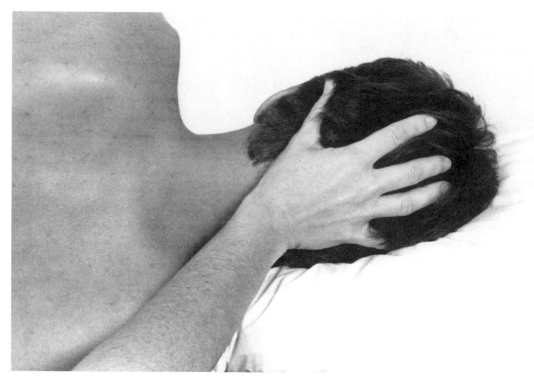

Figure 113: Hand position on the head for balancing of the dural tube. The base of the occiput is cradled in the palm of your hand while your fingers lay gently on the back of the head.

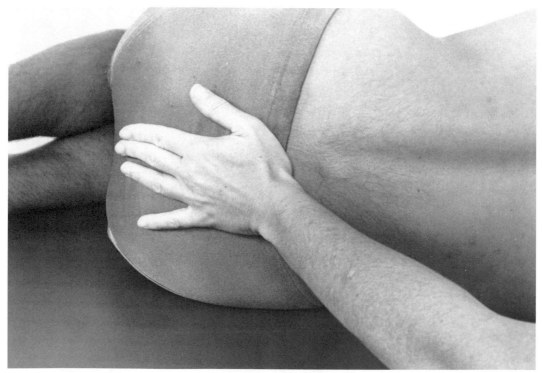

Figure 114: Hand position on the sacrum for balancing of the dural tube. The heel of your hand is in firm contact with the sacrum, while your fingers are in firm but light contact with the buttocks.

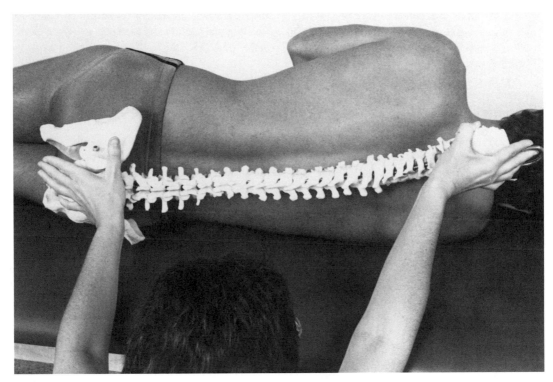

Figure 115: Balancing of the dural tube in the side-lying position.

A. Hand positions on a skeleton placed over the patient's body for balancing the dural tube in the side-lying position.

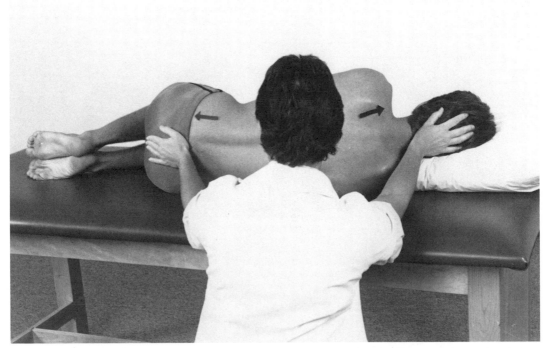

B. Apply the initial stretch of the dural tube by gently pushing the head and sacrum forward and then following the inherent tissue motion until it stops, then resumes a rhythmic rocking.

would for any other release sequence. When no further releases are felt or when the spontaneous movement ceases, again push forward gently on the occiput and sacrum and then pull gently back in a rocking motion (Fig. 116) until a regular rhythm is established. Once the rhythm is regular, the release is complete and you can remove your hands.

Never leave your patient with an irregular rhythm. If the sacrum and occiput are not rocking forward and backward in synchrony, repeat the above procedure until the rocking is symmetrical. When you have completed balancing the dural tube, return to whatever releases that were previously incomplete and repeat them.

If you have a patient who is unable to assume the side-lying position comfortably, the dural tube can be balanced with the person prone (Fig. 117), although passive maximum stretch of the dural tube is not possible in this position. The sitting position can also be used (Fig. 118) even though the sacrum is relatively fixed by this position.

Releasing the Dural Tube: Two-Person Technique

The two-person technique for releasing the dural tube can focus entirely on the dural tube, or a pelvic floor release and a thoracic inlet release can be performed simultaneously, depending upon the skills of the therapists. Have your patient lying supine in the hook-lying position (Fig. 119). Ask your patient to lift up his hips so you can slip your hand between his legs, and place your hand firmly on the sacrum, hooking your fingers over the rim of the pelvis on either side of the spinal column (Fig. 120). As your patient again lowers his hips to the plinth, apply traction to the sacrum. Have your patient straighten his legs while you rest on your elbow, while leaning backward to maintain your traction (Fig. 121). Rest your other hand just above your patient's pubis symphysis in proper position for a pelvic floor release (Fig. 122).

While all of this is happening, the therapist who is at the patient's head should be applying gentle cervical traction (Figs. 37-40). The more sensitive therapist should act as leader. If both therapists are equally sensitive, the one at the patient's head takes command. Any of the previously described variations of stretching the posterior cervical musculature can be used. In addition, a thoracic inlet release can be performed at the same time (Fig. 123).

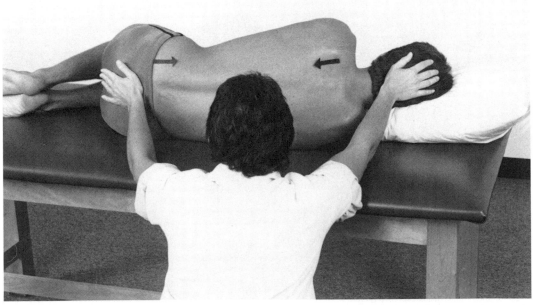

Figure 116: Recheck balance of the dural tube by gently pulling the head and sacrum into extension, again following the inherent tissue motion until it stops, then resume a rhythmic rocking.

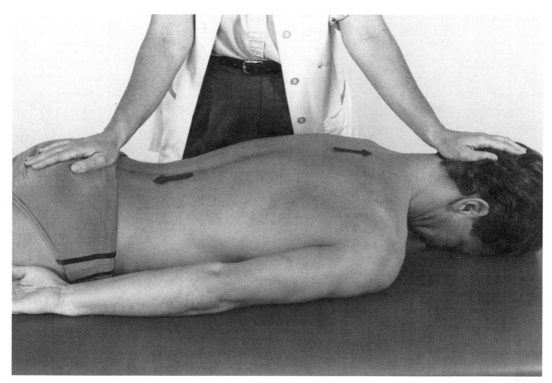

Figure 117: Balancing of the dural tube, with the patient prone.

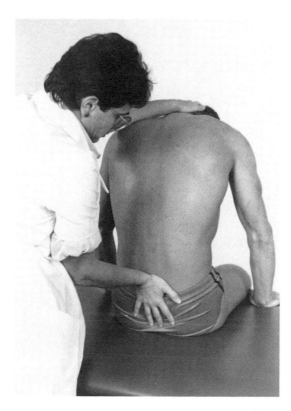

Figure 118: Balancing of the dural tube, with the patient sitting.

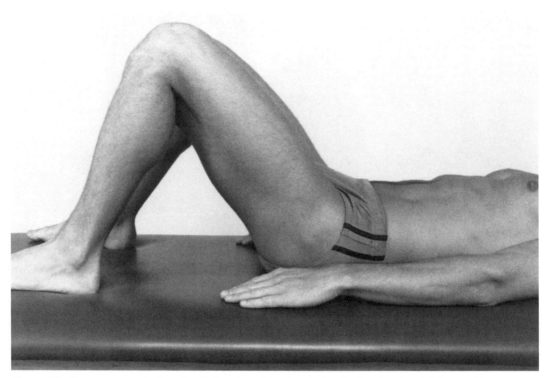

Figure 119: Two-person technique for balancing of the dural tube. Patient in a hook-lying position.

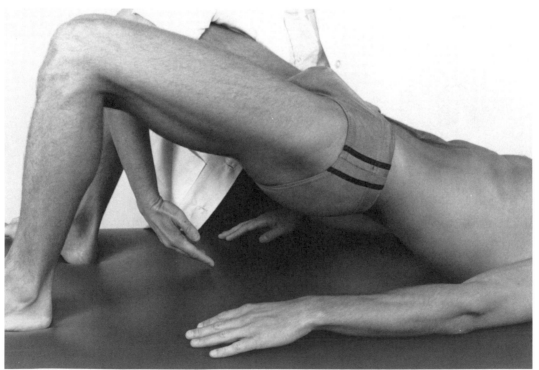

Figure 120: Two-person technique for balancing of the dural tube.

A-D. As the patient assumes the body bridge position, the therapist reaches between his legs to place a hand on his sacrum.

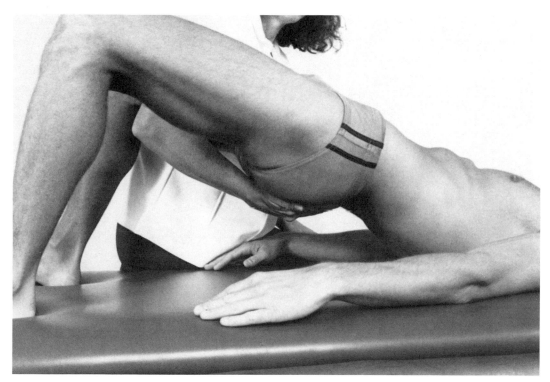

B. Two-person technique for balancing of the dural tube.

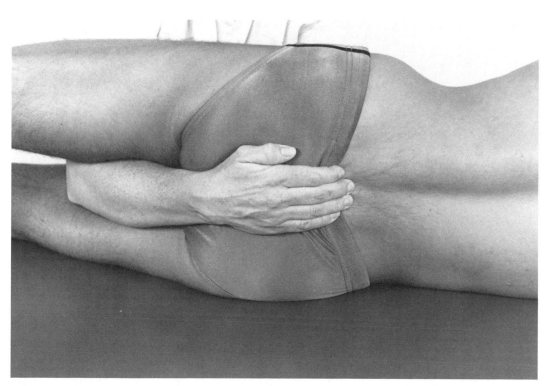

C. Hand position on the sacrum.

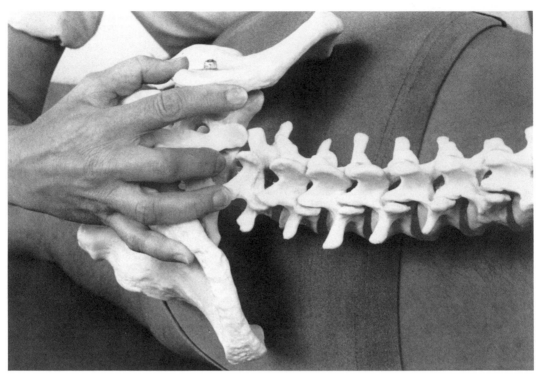

D. Hand position on a skeleton in position on the patient.

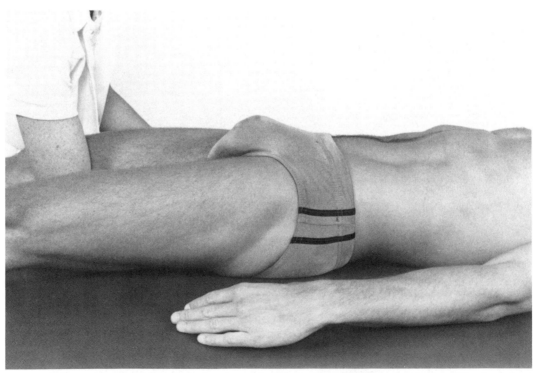

Figure 121: Two-person technique for balancing of the dural tube. Therapist and patient position to distract the sacrum during dural tube balancing.

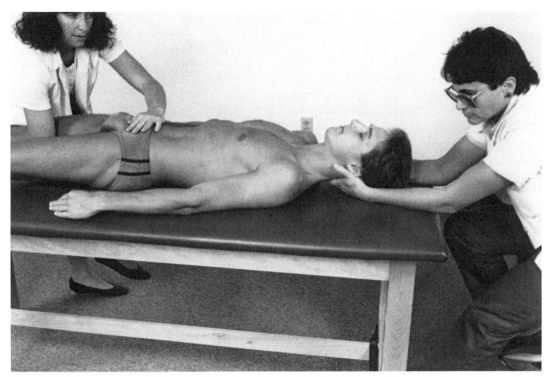

Figure 122: Two-person technique for balancing of the dural tube. Patient and therapists in position to begin balancing of the dural tube while performing a pelvic floor release.

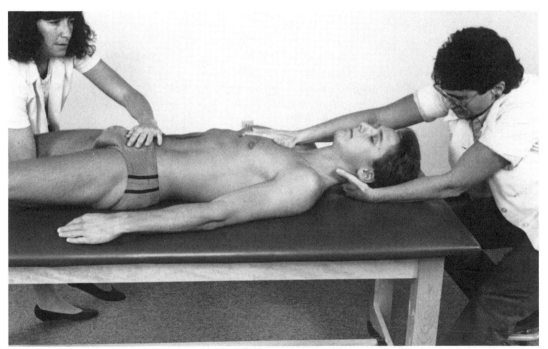

Figure 123: Two-person technique for balancing of the dural tube. Patient and therapists in position to begin balancing of the dural tube while performing a pelvic floor release and a thoracic inlet release.

The Initial Assessment

In addition to the usual assessment a therapist might perform for a given diagnosis, a detailed postural assessment must be done when considering myofascial treatment. While performing this assessment, as when performing any assessment, the therapist must be alert to signs and symptoms that do not correspond to the usual picture presented by a given complaint or diagnosis.[97] Assessment is never completed and constantly modifies the treatment given.

Because myofascial treatment results in postural change, the postural assessment should be very detailed so that you can document change in your clinical notes, in your reports to doctors, insurance companies, and lawyers, and, most importantly, in your discussions with your patients. The patient very frequently cannot detect changes with any degree of accuracy, especially during the initial stages of treatment when the changes may be so slight as to be not readily noticeable to the untrained eye. This is where documentation can be very useful. The final reason for complete documentation, of course, is that it allows you to monitor whether your treatment is causing change and to determine whether the change is in the proper direction.

When posture is being changed, the central nervous system is being re-educated to the new feelings that go with the improved body alignment. This initially causes a conflict between what the nervous system has become adjusted to and accepts as normal and the improved alignment, which the nervous system interprets as improper. Furthermore, the new transitional alignment may, in fact, be less stable than the old improper alignment. Both the conflict and the temporarily decreased stability may make your patient uncomfortable to the point of increased pain. If this happens, the postural changes need to be pointed out to your patient. This will help to reassure your patient that the changes are towards improvement and that, as his body adjusts, he will feel better.

The written assessment may be confusing to your patient. Therefore, for both my benefit and my patient's, I always take photographs at the first visit and periodically thereafter. All four postural views are taken, with the patient wearing minimal clothing. These photographs and the negatives are kept in the patient's file. The photographs are mounted, dated, and labeled whether pre- or post-treatment.

Quantifying a postural assessment is difficult since you do not want to be standing close to your patient with goniometer, plumb bob, and ruler in hand. Estimates with periodic measurements should be sufficient, once you have measured enough to calibrate your eye. Standard range of motion measurements should also be part of the overall assessment. The assessment forms which follow (Appendix) give the broad outline of the evaluation process that I use. At times, greater or lesser detail is noted, depending upon the patient's initial complaint and the complexity of his problem. If you choose to photocopy and use the following forms, be sure to indicate the degree of deviation when, for example, one shoulder is higher than the other.

One advantage of using assessment forms is that, at a minimum, all of the items on them are assessed periodically. That way, the same items can be noted and change can be documented when progress notes are written for the physician, insurance company, or attorney. All therapists know well the frustration of sitting down to write a report and finding inconsistent use of specific measures. My frustration is kept to a minimum by the use of assessment forms. I also use flow sheets composed on the computer to speed up writing progress letters and to facilitate following change. After each re-evaluation, the latest changes are entered on a flow sheet; when the flow sheet is filled, it is printed and placed in the patient's chart. The chart is then flagged for a progress letter. That way, the referring doctor is kept current of changes and will know that progress is being made with the patient. Justification of recertification for Medicare purposes are handled quite easily this way. The flow sheet is also a very useful way to educate physicians as to what myofascial treatment can do for their other patients. Education of physicians is, of course, very important whether you live in a state which allows physical therapy without physician referral or only with physician referral.

The first part of the initial visit is spent taking the patient's history with as much detail as he feels is necessary. Sometimes I tape this history on my dictaphone and other times I take notes. If I tape the history, then I have the history transcribed and kept as part of the chart. If the initial injury was due to an accident, the history may be an important aid in determining which joints may have been tractioned, compressed, or pushed beyond their physiologic range, all of which can lead to twisting of the body. Initial treatment is directed toward these joints until the myofascial feedback begins to guide the treatment.

The history is placed at the back of the chart and I usually do not look at it again until I am ready to dictate a progress note or discharge letter. The same is true for any notes that I may take. Why bother to listen to the patient's story then? I listen for the very simple reason that the patient needs to tell it and the telling allows a rapport to develop between us. While the story ("I was in a car accident") is being told, I attempt to extract facts such as "I was thrown to the left" or "my head hit the roof." The reality is that my postural assessment is more important than the patient's story in my decision about where to begin treatment. However, should treatment evolve into a somato-emotional release, this background information can help me anticipate what types of physical movement may occur.

The second part of the initial visit is the postural assessment. It is performed as a strictly hands-off visual inspection. I take the photographs at the beginning of the assessment, when the patient is holding to his best posture. I then note during the assessment whether the posture changes as the patient relaxes. The major change that is likely to occur is usually in trunk rotation. I like to dictate this part of the evaluation and mark the assessment forms later. Dictation serves three purposes. First, it is faster for me than marking the forms. Second, a secretary can listen to the dictation, mark the forms, and add in any additional comments I made at the time. Needless to say, having the forms on the computer is the most efficient method for record keeping, but photocopied forms work nearly as well. Third, during dictation, the patient's posture is called to his attention by hearing the various landmarks from which I monitored change. When the patient later looks in the mirror, he also sees change and progress. This helps make the patient more of a participant and less of a subject. Many times, a patient will come in eager to report a new change in posture and resulting physical sensation since the last visit in almost a game of "I saw it first!"

The postural assessment as listed on the forms is quite straightforward. Ask your patient to stand with his back to a wall and his feet several inches away from the wall without being very specific as to how far away. The patient with balance problems, spatial orientation problems, or body image problems will be closer to the wall and may even lean against it. Without being judgmental, ask him to move away from the wall and make a silent note of this behavior. Later, you will be able to decide why your patient stood this way. He may merely have misunderstood your directions.

Always have your patient face you first so that you tell your patient nonverbally that you will never talk behind his back. Ask your patient to focus on a spot over your head. I am always seated during the postural assessment so that my patients do not have to tilt their heads to look over mine. I prefer to do the postural assessment with patients not wearing glasses. Removing the glasses allows their eyes to be seen clearly. It also allows balance disturbances to be detected that are being compensated by vision. If removing the glasses is not possible because taking them off is too stressful in terms of focus or balance disturbance, then ask your patient to remove his glasses only until you have completed the facial part of the assessment. Before beginning to dictate, also ask your patients to push their hair away from their ears and away from the back of their necks. You do not want a patient to hold his hair with a hand, since this alone changes posture.

At the completion of the postural assessment, if the patient has not been standing with his feet parallel, but with his trunk rotated, ask him to stand with his feet parallel while facing you. Always stand close to the patient when you ask this, because many patients lose their balance when asked to stand this way. If standing with feet parallel does not cause a balance loss, then you can move away and visually inspect again. By asking that the feet be parallel, any rotation will be exaggerated and confirmed. Do not ask a patient to hold this position for long because he is liable to feel very uncomfortable and become very irritable quickly. Specifying a particular stance is perceived as a criticism of his posture either consciously or subconsciously.

Once having completed the postural evaluation, skin mobility can then be assessed with the patient in the standing position. Skin mobility can also be assessed with the patient sitting or lying down. Scars are always palpated for restriction during this part of the assessment.

Following skin mobility assessment, spinal movement and sacro-iliac movement should be assessed in the standing position.[98] First, assess visually before palpating the movement. The most important aspect is the quality of movement. Symmetry and asymmetry of movement need to be noted. Generally, symmetry allows the most energy-efficient movement patterns or the best compensation available for limited movement. Rarely, if ever, is a pathological condition symmetrical. The patient will often perform a motion without movement occurring at the proper spinal segments. Much important information is lost if only quantity of movement is noted. Immobility and hypermobility must be localized to vertebral level. Most therapists are accustomed to doing this in the lumbar area, but neglect doing it in the thoracic and cervical areas. Spinal and sacro-iliac movement should be reassessed with the patient sitting to identify any effect of tight leg musculature on the pelvis. Thus, the evaluation process is a systematic approach that will identify restricted myofascial structures and guide your initial treatment approach.

The myofascial restrictions identified in this manner are only the most obvious and most superficial in terms of effect on the entire body. What is identified in the initial assessment will ultimately not be found to be the key restricted structures. Keep in mind that the body is a kinetic chain. A change in the ability to move in any part of the body affects the ability to move every other part of the body. Postural malalignment in any part of the body causes postural malalignment throughout the entire body.

The most dramatic illustration of the effects of one part of the body on all other parts is the patient with a flaccid paralysis due to peripheral nerve injury caused by disease or an accident. The entire body must adjust to the passive malposition. In contrast, spastic paralysis dynamically causes malposition. While the presence of both of these problems makes myofascial treatment less efficient and beneficial, neither is a contra-indication to myofascial stretching. In fact, myofascial stretching is the safest method of stretching in the presence of flaccid paralysis because the feedback from the patient's body will prevent over-stretching and will, thus, allow protective tightness to remain.

Once the standing and sitting evaluations are completed, the supine evaluation is performed. Actual measurement of leg length must be performed from whatever reproducible landmark with which you are comfortable. Remember that many leg length discrepancies are due to pelvic twisting. A leg length discrepancy reaching back into childhood can still be changed with myofascial stretching. Anatomic changes cannot be overcome, but the soft tissue response to them may be changeable.

Conclusion

This manual is only an introduction to the concept of myofascial release. The key to myofascial release is the sensitivity of the therapist's hands. The only way to develop and refine this skill is to place your hands on as many different people as possible to learn the feel of the soft tissues and their inherent motion. Next, you must learn to trust what you are feeling through your hands and respond to those feelings. Allow your patients to lead you and direct treatment. Above all, become comfortable with yourself, be relaxed, and allow yourself to explore alternative ways to relate to your patients and respond to their needs.

Appendix
EVALUATION FORM
Visual Postural Assessment

STANDING

I. Facing Forward

Head Tilt
- neutral
- left
- right

Head Rotation
- neutral
- left
- right

Facial Crease
- equal
- deeper left
- deeper right

Eyes
- level
- left higher
- right higher
- equal size
- left bigger
- right bigger

Mouth
- symmetrical
- left longer
- right longer
- not pulled
- pulled left
- pulled right
- level
- left elevated
- right elevated

Nose
- midline
- deviated left
- deviated right

Ears
- level
- left elevated
- right elevated
- neutral
- left externally rotated
- right externally rotated
- left internally rotated
- right internally rotated

Neck
- equal length
- left longer
- right longer

Shoulders
- equal length
- left longer
- right longer
- level
- left elevated
- right elevated
- neutral
- left protracted
- right protracted
- left retracted
- right retracted

Arms
- neutral
- left external rotation
- right external rotation
- left internal rotation
- right internal rotation
- equal length
- left longer
- right longer
- equal abduction
- left greater abduction
- right greater abduction

Trunk
- neutral
- shifted left
- shifted right
- equal length
- left longer
- right longer
- equal creases
- left higher
- right higher
- left longer
- right longer
- neutral
- rotated left
- rotated right

Pelvis
- level
- left higher
- right higher
- neutral
- left retracted
- right retracted
- left protracted
- right protracted

Thighs
neutral
left external rotation
right external rotation
left internal rotation
right internal rotation

Knees
level
left higher
right higher
equal
left recurvatum
right recurvatum
left flexed
right flcxed

Lower Leg
neutral
left varus
right varus
left valgus
right valgus

Foot
neutral left
neutral right
pronated left
pronated left
inverted left
inverted right

Forefoot
neutral left
neutral right
left varus
right varus
left valgus
right valgus

Weight Bearing
equal
greater left
greater right

II. Facing Right

Head
neutral
forward head posture
hyperextended

Ear
over acromium
forward of acromium
behind acromium

Shoulder
over hip
forward of hip
behind hip
neutral
protracted
retracted

Hip
over middle of knee joint
forward of knee joint
behind knee joint
neutral
protracted
retracted
over malleolus
forward of malleolus
behind malleolus

Knee
neutral
flexed
recurvatum
over malleolus
forward of malleolus
behind malleolus

Cervical Lordosis
WNL
exaggerated
flattened
equals lumbar lordosis
greater than lumbar lordosis
less than lumbar lordosis

Thoracic Kyphosis
WNL
exaggerated
flattened

Lumbar Lordosis
WNL
exaggerated
flattened

III. Facing Backwards

Head Tilt
neutral
left
right

Head Rotation
neutral
left
right

Ears
level
left elevated
right elevated
neutral
left externally rotated
right externally rotated
left internally rotated
right internally rotated

Neck
equal length
left longer
right longer

Shoulders
equal length
left longer
right longer
level
left elevated
right elevated
neutral
left protracted
right protracted
left retracted
right retracted

Arms
neutral
left external rotation
right external rotation
left internal rotation
right internal rotation
equal length
left longer
right longer
equal abduction
left greater abduction
right greater abduction

Trunk
neutral
shifted left
shifted right
equal length
left longer

right longer
equal creases
left higher
right higher
left longer
right longer
neutral
rotated left
rotated right

Pelvis
level
left higher
right higher
neutral
left retracted
right retracted
left protracted
right protracted

Thighs
neutral
left external rotation
right external rotation
left internal rotation
right internal rotation

Knees
level
left higher
right higher
equal
left recurvatum
right recurvatum
left flexed
right flexed

Lower Leg
neutral
left varus
right varus
left valgus
right valgus

Foot
neutral left
neutral right
pronated left
pronated right
inverted left
inverted right

Weight Bearing
equal
greater left
greater right

IV. Facing Left
  Head
    neutral
    forward head posture
    hyperextended
  Ear
    over acromium
    forward of acromium
    behind acromium
  Shoulder
    over hip
    forward of hip
    behind hip
    neutral
    protracted
    retracted
  Hip
    over middle of knee joint
    forward of knee joint
    behind knee joint
    neutral
    protracted
    retracted
    over malleolus
    forward of malleolus
    behind malleolus

  Knee
    neutral
    flexed
    recurvatum
    over malleolus
    forward of malleolus
    behind malleolus
  Cervical Lordosis
    WNL
    exaggerated
    flattened
    equals lumbar lordosis
    greater than lumbar lordosis
    less than lumbar lordosis
  Thoracic Kyphosis
    WNL
    exaggerated
    flattened
  Lumbar Lordosis
    WNL
    exaggerated
    flattened

SITTING
I. Facing Forward
  Head Tilt
    neutral
    left
    right
  Head Rotation
    neutral
    left
    right
  Facial Crease
    equal
    deeper left
    deeper right
  Eyes
    level
    left higher
    right higher
    equal size
    left bigger
    right bigger
  Mouth
    symmetrical
    left longer
    right longer
    not pulled
    pulled left
    pulled right
    level
    left elevated
    right elevated

  Nose
    midline
    deviated left
    deviated right
  Ears
    level
    left elevated
    right elevated
    neutral
    left externally rotated
    right externally rotated
    left internally rotated
    right internally rotated
  Neck
    equal length
    left longer
    right longer
  Shoulders
    equal length
    left longer
    right longer
    level
    left elevated
    right elevated
    neutral
    left protracted
    right protracted
    left retracted
    right retracted

Arms
  neutral
  left external rotation
  right external rotation
  left internal rotation
  right internal rotation
  equal length
  left longer
  right longer
  equal abduction
  left greater abduction
  right greater abduction

Trunk
  neutral
  shifted left
  shifted right
  equal length
  left longer
  right longer
  equal creases

II. Facing Right
Head
  neutral
  forward head posture
  hyperextended
Ear
  over acromium
  forward of acromium
  behind acromium
Shoulder
  over hip
  forward of hip
  behind hip
  neutral
  protracted
  retracted

III. Facing Backwards
Head Tilt
  neutral
  left
  right
Head Rotation
  neutral
  left
  right
Ears
  level
  left elevated
  right elevated
  neutral
  left externally rotated
  right externally rotated
  left internally rotated
  right internally rotated

  left higher
  right higher
  left longer
  right longer
  neutral
  rotated left
  rotated right
Pelvis
  level
  left higher
  right higher
  neutral
  left retracted
  right retracted
  left protracted
  right protracted

Cervical Lordosis
  WNL
  exaggerated
  flattened
  equals lumbar lordosis
  greater than lumbar lordosis
  less than lumbar lordosis
Thoracic Kyphosis
  WNL
  exaggerated
  flattened
Lumbar Lordosis
  WNL
  exaggerated
  flattened

Neck
  equal length
  left longer
  right longer
Shoulders
  equal length
  left longer
  right longer
  level
  left elevated
  right elevated
  neutral
  left protracted
  right protracted
  left retracted
  right retracted

Arms
- neutral
- left external rotation
- right external rotation
- left internal rotation
- right internal rotation
- equal length
- left longer
- right longer
- equal abduction
- left greater abduction
- right greater abduction

Trunk
- neutral
- shifted left
- shifted right
- equal length
- left longer
- right longer

- equal creases
- left higher
- right higher
- left longer
- right longer
- neutral
- rotated left
- rotated right

Pelvis
- level
- left higher
- right higher
- neutral
- left retracted
- right retracted
- left protracted
- right protracted

IV. Facing Left

Head
- neutral
- forward head posture
- hyperextended

Ear
- over acromium
- forward of acromium
- behind acromium

Shoulder
- over hip
- forward of hip
- behind hip
- neutral
- protracted
- retracted

Cervical Lordosis
- WNL
- exaggerated
- flattened
- equals lumbar lordosis
- greater than lumbar lordosis
- less than lumbar lordosis

Thoracic Kyphosis
- WNL
- exaggerated
- flattened

Lumbar Lordosis
- WNL
- exaggerated
- flattened

Analysis of Movement

STANDING

I. Cervical

Rotation Left	Full	3/4	1/2	1/4	1/8	0
Rotation Right	Full	3/4	1/2	1/4	1/8	0
Lateral Flexion Left	Full	3/4	1/2	1/4	1/8	0
Lateral Flexion Right	Full	3/4	1/2	1/4	1/8	0

Forward Flexion   Chin touches

               chest   1 finger   2 fingers

3 fingers   4 fingers   minimal   0

Hyperextension	Full	3/4	1/2	1/4	1/8	0

II. Thoracic and Lumbar

Forward Flexion — fingertips to:

                floor   top of foot   ankle

       above ankle   mid calf   middle of knee

            mid thigh   hip joints

smooth symmetrical thoracic curve   asymmetrical thoracic curve

   flattened   sharply angled apex_____

   immobile segments _____

   hypermobile segments _____

smooth reversal lumbar lordotic curve   flattened low back

   immobile segments _____

   hypermobile segments _____

Left Lateral Flexion—fingertips to:

                floor   top of foot   ankle

       above ankle   mid calf   middle of knee

            mid thigh   hip joints

smooth symmetrical thoracic curve   asymmetrical thoracic curve

   flattened   sharply angled apex_____

   immobile segments _____

   hypermobile segments _____

smooth lumbar curve right   flat lumbar curve right

   immobile segments _____

   hypermobile segments _____

Right Lateral Flexion—fingertips to:

                floor   top of foot   ankle

       above ankle   mid calf   middle of knee

            mid thigh   hip joints

smooth symmetrical thoracic curve   asymmetrical thoracic curve

   flattened   sharply angled apex _____

   immobile segments _____

   hypermobile segments _____

smooth reversal lumbar lordotic curve   flattened low back

   immobile segments _____

   hypermobile segments _____

Hyperextension

full range of motion	3/4	1/2	1/4	1/8	0

   smooth curve   asymmetrical   fulcrum at _____

   immobile segments _____

   hypermobile segments _____

III. Legs

Squat Test   both heels on floor to end range

left heel on floor to end range   left heel lifts

right heel on floor to end range   right heel lifts

SITTING

I. Forward Flexion

smooth symmetrical thoracic curve   asymmetrical thoracic curve

flattened   sharply angled apex _____

immobile segments _____

hypermobile segments _____

smooth reversal lumbar lordotic curve   flattened low back

immobile segments _____

hypermobile segments _____

Left Lateral Flexion

smooth symmetrical thoracic curve   asymmetrical thoracic curve

flattened   sharply angled apex _____

immobile segments _____

hypermobile segments _____

smooth lumbar curve right   flat lumbar curve right

immobile segments _____

hypermobile segments _____

Right Lateral Flexion

smooth symmetrical thoracic curve   asymmetrical thoracic curve

flattened   sharply angled apex _____

immobile segments _____

hypermobile segments _____

smooth lumbar curve left   flat lumbar curve left

immobile segments _____

hypermobile segments _____

Hyperextension

full range of motion   3/4   1/2   1/4   1/8   0

smooth curve   assymmetrical   fulcrum at _____

immobile segments _____

hypermobile segments _____

Palpation

STANDING

I. Skin Mobility

Anterior Chest Wall Tightness

upward	downward	left	right

Anterior Abdominal Wall Tightness

upward	downward	left	right

Upper Thoracic Tightness

upward	downward	left	right

Lower Thoracic Tightness

upward	downward	left	right

Lumbar Tightness

upward	downward	left	right

II. Anterior Superior Iliac Crests

equal	left higher	right higher
	left lower	right lower
neutral	left rotated up	right rotated up
	left rotated down	right rotated down

III. Posterior Superior Iliac Crests

equal	left higher	right higher
	left lower	right lower
neutral	left rotated up	right rotated up
	left rotated down	right rotated down

SUPINE

I. Skin Mobility

Anterior Chest Wall Tightness

upward	downward	left	right

Anterior Abdominal Wall Tightness

upward	downward	left	right

II. Anterior Superior Iliac Crests

equal	left higher	right higher
	left lower	right lower
neutral	left rotated up	right rotated up
	left rotated down	right rotated down

III. Pubic Tubercles

equal	left higher	right higher
	left lower	right lower
neutral	left rotated up	right rotated up
	left rotated down	right rotated down

IV. Leg Lengths

left medial malleolus higher	right medial malleolus higher
left medial malleolus lower	right medial malleolus lower
measured leg lengths	equal unequal _____

V. Leg Position — with hip and knee extended

rotation	left neutral			right neutral		
left external rotation	full	3/4	1/2	1/4	0	
right external rotation	full	3/4	1/2	1/4	0	
left internal rotation	full	3/4	1/2	1/4	0	
right internal rotation	full	3/4	1/2	1/4	0	

abduction/adduction   left neutral   right neutral
   left abduction _____   right abduction _____
   left adduction _____   right adduction _____

VI. Active Range of Motion Measurements — note pain with movement

	left	right
Cervical		
rotation		
lateral flexion		
Shoulder		
flexion		
external rotation		
internal rotation		
abduction		
Knee		
flexion with 90 degrees hip flexion		
extension with 90 degrees hip flexion		
Hip		
flexion with free knee flexion		
extension with 90 degree knee flexion		
external rotaion		
internal rotation		
abduction		
adduction		

PRONE

I. Skin Mobility

Upper Thoracic Tightness
   upward   downward   left   right
Lower Thoracic Tightness
   upward   downward   left   right

Lumbar Tightness
   upward   downward   left   right

III. Posterior Superior Iliac Crests

equal   left higher   right higher
                        left lower   right lower
neutral   left rotated up   right rotated up
                        left rotated down   right rotated down

III. Sacral Sulci

equal   left higher   right higher
left lower   right lower

IV. Sacral Tuberous Ligament

equal   left higher   right higher
left lower   right lower

V. Gluteal Cleft

midline   deviated left   deviated right

References

1. Upledger JE, Vredevoogd JD: Craniosacral Therapy. Seattle WA, Eastland Press, 1983.

2. Manheim CJ, Lavett DK: The Self-Healing Body: Craniosacral Therapy and Somato-emotional Release. Thorofare, NJ, Slack, Inc., 1989.

3. Manheim CJ, Lavett DK: Somato-emotional Release and the Chronic Pain State. To be published.

4. Cailliet R: Soft Tissue Pain and Disability. Philadelphia, FA Davis Company, 1977.

5. Barnes JF: Course Notes: Myofascial Release Seminar I. Houston, Tx., 1985.

6. Barnes JF: Course Notes: Intermediate Myofascial Release II and Cranio-Sacral Therapy Seminar. Captiva Island, Fl., 1986.

7. Barnes JF: Course Notes: Somato-emotional Release Seminar. Hilton Head Island, S.C., 1986.

8. Garfin SR, Tipton CM, Mubarek SJ, et al: Role of fascia in maintenance of muscle tension and pressure. J Appl Physiol, 1981; 51:317-320.

9. Hollinshead WH: Functional Anatomy of the Limbs and Back, ed 2. Philadelphia, WB Saunders Company, 1960.

10. Schaeffer JP (ed): Morris' Human Anatomy, ed 11. New York, McGraw-Hill Book Company, Inc, 1953.

11. Hoppenfeld S, Hutton R: Physical Examination of the Spine and Extremities. New York, Appleton-Century-Crofts, 1976.

12. Maitland GD: Vertebral Manipulation. London, Butterworth & Company, Ltd, 1986.

13. Ebner, M: Connective Tissue Massage: Theory and Therapeutic Application. Huntington, New York, Robert E. Krieger Publishing Company, 1962.

14. Bonica JJ: Management of myofascial pain syndromes in general practice. JAMA, 1957; 164:732-738.

15. Campbell SM: Is the tender point concept valid? Am J Med, 1986; 81(3):33-37.

16. Eisenberg D, Wright TL: Encounters with Qi: Exploring Chinese Medicine. New York, Norton, 1985.

17. Gorrell RL: Musculofascial pain: Treatment by local injection of analgesic drugs. JAMA, 1950; 142:557-561.

18. Grosshandler S, Stratas NE, Toomey TC, et al: Chronic neck and shoulder pain. Focusing on myofascial origins. Postgrad Med, 1985; 77:149-158.

19. Jaeger B, Reeves JL: Quantification of changes in myofascial trigger point sensitivity with the pressure algometer following passive stretch. Pain, 1986; 27:203-210.

20. Reynolds MD: Myofascial trigger points in persistent posttraumatic shoulder pain. South Med J, 1984; 77:1277-1280.

21. Russell J, Vipraio GA, Morgan WW, et al: Is there a metabolic basis for the fibrositis syndrome? Am J Med, 1986; 81:50-54.

22. Simons DG: Fibrositis/fibromyalgia: A form of myofascial trigger points? Am J Med, 1986; 81:93-98.

23. Simons DG: Myofascial pain syndrome due to trigger points. International Rehabilitation Medicine Association Monograph Series, 1987; 1:1-39.

24. Slocumb JC: Neurological factors in chronic pelvic pain: Trigger points and the abdominal pelvic pain syndrome. Am J Obstet Gynecol, 1984; July:536-543.

25. Travell JG, Simons DG: Myofascial Pain and Dysfunction: The Trigger Point Manual. Baltimore, William & Wilkins, 1983.

26. Tunks E, Crook J, Norman G, et al: Tender points in fibromyalgia. Pain, 1988; 34:11-19.
    Yunus M, Masi AT, Feigenbaum SL, et al: Primary fibromyalgia (fibrositis): Clinical study of 50 patients with matched normal controls. Semin Arthritis Rheum, 1981; 11:151-171.

28. Inman VT, Saunders JBDM: Referred pain from skeletal structures. J Nerv Men Dis, 1944; 99:660-667.

29. Bates T, Grunwaldt E: Myofascial pain in childhood. J Pediatr, 1958; 53:198-209.

30. Grosshandler S, Burney R: The myofascial syndrome. NC Med J, 1979; 40:562-565.

31. Hockaday JM, Whitty CWM: Patterns of referred pain in the normal subject. Brain, 1967; 90:481-496.

32. Jaeger B: Myofascial referred pain patterns: The role of trigger points. Journal of the California Dental Association, 1985; 13:27-28.

33. Kellgren JH: A preliminary account of referred pains arising from muscle. Br Med J, 1938; 1:325-327.

34. Kleier DJ: Referred pain from a myofascial trigger point mimicking pain of endodontic origin. Journal of Endodontics, 1985; 11:408-411.

35. Lewis T, Kellgren JH: Observations relating to referred pain, visceromotor reflexes and other associated phenomena. Clin Sci, 1939; 1:47-71.

36. Melzack R, Stillwell DM, Fox EJ: Trigger points and acupuncture points for pain: Correlations and implications. Pain, 1977; 3:3-23.

37. Pace JB: Commonly overlooked pain syndromes responsive to simple therapy. Postgrad Med, 1975; 58:107-113.

38. Schwartz RG, Gall NG, Grant AE: Abdominal pain in quadriparesis: Myofascial syndrome as unsuspected cause. Arch Phys Med Rehabil, 1984; 65:44-46.

39. Simons DG, Travell JG: Myofascial origins of low back pain: I: Principles of diagnosis and treatment. Postgrad Med, 1983; 73:66-77.

40. Simons, DG, Travell JG: Myofascial origins of low back pain: II: Torso muscles. Postgrad Med, 1983; 73:81-92.

41. Simons DG, Travell JG: Myofascial origins of low back pain: III: Pelvic and lower extremity muscles. Postgrad Med, 1983; 73:99-108.

42. Sola AE, Kuitert JH: Myofascial trigger point pain in the neck and shoulder girdle. Northwest Medicine, 1955; 980-984.

43. Travell JG: Temporomandibular joint pain referred from muscles of the head and neck. J Prosthe Dent, 1960; 10:745-763.

44. Travell JG: Identification of myofascial trigger point syndromes: A case of atypical facial neuralgia. Arch Phys Med Rehabil, 1981; 62:100-106.

45. Travell JG, Rinzler SH: The myofascial genesis of pain. Postgrad Med, 1952; 11:425-434.

46. Wyant GM: Chronic pain syndromes and their treatment. Trigger points. Canadian Anaesthesiology Society Journal, 1979; 26:216-219.

47. Butler JH, Folke LEA, Bandt CL: A descriptive survey of signs and symptoms associated with the myofascial pain-dysfunction syndrome. J Am Den Assoc, 1975; 90:635-639.

48. Fricton JR, Auvinen, MD, Dykstra D, et al: Myofascial pain syndrome: Electromyographic changes associated with local twitch response. Arch Phys Med Rehabil, 1985; 66:314-317.

49. Lewit K, Simons DG: Myofascial pain: Relief by post-isometric relaxation. Arch Phys Med Rehabil, 1984; 65:452-456.

50. MacDonald AJR: Abnormally tender muscle regions and associated painful movements. Pain, 1980; 8:197-205.

51. Coulehan J: Primary fibromyalgia. Am Fam Physician, 1985; 32:170-177.

52. Leandrim M, Brunetti O, Parodi, CI: Teletthermographic findings after transcutaneous electrical nerve stimulation. Phys Ther, 1986; 66:210-213.

53. Sheon RP: Regional myofascial pain and the fibrositis syndrome (fibromyalgia). Compr Ther, 1986; 12:42-52.

54. Snyder-Mackler L, Bork C, Bourbon B, et al: Effect of helium-neon laser on musculoskeletal trigger points. Phys Ther, 1986; 66:1087-1090.

55. Wolfe F: Development of criteria for the diagnosis of fibrositis. Am J Med, 1986; 81:99-104.

56. Campbell SM, Bennett RM: Fibrositis. Disease a Month, 1986; 32:653-722.

57. Schmalbruch H: Contracture knots in normal and diseased muscle fibres. Brain, 1973; 96:637-640.

58. Simons DG: Muscle pain syndromes. Am J Phys Med, Part I, 54:289-311, 1975. Part II, 55:15-42, 1976.

59. Dexter JR, Simons DG: Local twitch response in human muscle evoked by palpation and needle penetration of a trigger point. Arch Phys Med Rehabil, 1981; 62:521.

60. Fricton JR, Kroening R, Haley D, et al: Myofascial pain syndrome of the head and neck: A review of clinical characteristics of 164 patients. Oral Surgery, 1985; 60:615-623.

61. Kine G, Warfield C: Myofascial pain syndrome. Hosp Prac, 1986; 21:194B-194C, 194G-194H.

62. Dittrich RJ: Low back pain—referred pain from deep somatic structure of the back. Lancet, 1953; 73:63-68.

64. Berges PU: Myofascial pain syndromes. Postgrad Med, 1973; 53:161-168.

65. Epstein SE, Gerber LH, Borer, JS: Chest wall syndrome. JAMA, 1979; 241:2793-2797.

66. Rinzler SH, Travell JG: Therapy directed at the somatic component of cardiac pain. Am Heart J, 1948; 35:248-268.

67. Rubin D: Myofascial trigger point syndromes: An approach to management. Arch Phys Med Rehabil, 1981; 62:107-110.

68. Ruskin AP: Facial neuralgia with trigger point on finger, one case suggesting a cortically mediated response. Arch Neurol, 1980; 37:672.

69. Travell JG: A trigger point for hiccup. J Am Osteopath Assoc, 1977; 77:308-312.

70. Fine PG: Myofascial trigger point pain in children. J Pediatr, 1987; 111:547-548.

71. Laskin DM: Etiology of the pain-dysfunction syndrome. J Am Dent Assoc, 1969; 79:147-153.

72. Graff-Radford SB, Jaeger B, Reeves JL: Myofascial pain may present clinically as occipital neuralgia. Neurosurgery, 1986; 19:610-613.

73. Schultz DR: Occipital neuralgia. J AM Osteopath Assoc, 1977; 76:335-343.

74. Weed ND: When shoulder pain isn't bursitis. Postgrad Med, 1983; 74:97-104.

75. Graff-Radford SB, Reeves JL, Jaeger B: Management of head and neck pain: Effectiveness of altering factors perpetuating myofascial pain. Postgrad Med, 1985; 77:149-158.

76. Travell JG: Rapid relief of acute "stiff neck" by ethyl chloride spray. J Am Medical Women's Association, 1949; 4:89-95.

77. Weeks VD, Travell JG: Postural vertigo due to trigger areas in the sternocleidomastoid muscle. J Pediatr, 1955; 47:315-327.

78. Lewit K: Postisometric relaxation in combination with other methods of muscular facilitation and inhibition. Manual Medicine, 1986; 2:101-104.

79. Brown BR: Diagnosis and therapy of common myofascial syndromes. JAMA, 1978; 239:646-648.

80. Gunn CC, Milbrandt WE: Shoulder pain, cervical spondylosis and acupuncture. American Journal of Acupuncture, 1977; 5:121-128.

81. Lewith GT, Machin D: A randomized trial to evaluate the effect of infra-red stimulation of local trigger points, versus placebo, on the pain caused by cervical osteoarthrosis. Acupunc Electro-ther Res, 1981; 6:277-284.

82. Waylonis GW: Long-term follow-up on patients with fibrositis treated with acupuncture. The Ohio State Medical Journal, 1977; 73(May):299-302.

83. Wyant GM: Chronic pain syndromes and their treatment. The piriformis syndrome. Canadian Anesthiology Society Journal, 1979; 26:305-308.

84. Brown BR: Myofascial and musculoskeletal pain. Int Anesthesiol Clin, 1983; 21:139-151.

85. Danneskiold-Samsoe B, Christiansen E, Lund B, et al: Regional muscle tension and pain ("fibrositis"): Effect of massage on myoglobin in plasma. Scand J Rehabil Med, 1983; 15:17-20.

86. Travell JG: Pain mechanisms in connective tissue, in Ragan, C (ed): Connective Tissues, Transactions of the Second Conference, May 24-25, 1951. New York, Josiah Macy Jr Foundation, 1952.

87. Barr ML, Kiernan JA: The Human Nervous System: Anatomical Viewpoint. Philadelphia, Harper & Row, 1983.

88. Brieg A: Biomechanics of the CNS: Some Basic Pathological Phenomena. Stockholm, Alquist & Wiksell, 1960.

89. Brieg A: Biomechanical considerations in the straight leg raising test. Spine, 1979; 4:242-250.

90. Brieg A, Marions O: Biomechanics of the lumbosacral nerve roots. Acta Radiol, 1963; 1:1141-1160.

91. Charnley J: Orthopaedic signs in the diagnosis of disc protrusion with special reference to the straight-leg-raising test. Lancet, 1951; 1:186-192.

92. Reid J: Ascending nerve roots and tightness of dura. NZ Med J, 1958; 57:16-26.

93. Frykholm R: Cervical epidural structures, periradicular and epineural sheath. Acta Chir Scand, 1951; 102:10-20.

94. Cyriax J: Textbook of Orthopaedic Medicine, vol 1, ed 7. London, Balliere Tindall, 1978.

95. Edgar M, Nundy S: Innervation of spinal dura mater. J Neurol Neurosurg Psychiatry, 1966; 29:530-534.

96. Massey AE: Movement of pain-sensitive structures in the neural canal, in Grieve GP, (ed): Modern Manual Treatment of The Vertebral Column. London, Churchill Livingston, 1986.

97. Tucker LE: Diagnosis: back pain of extraspinal origin. Hospital Medicine, 1981; April.

98. Rex LH: Introduction to muscle energy technique. URSA Foundation Course Notes. 1987.

99. Hallin RP: Sciatic pain and the piriformis muscle. Postgrad Med, 1983; 74:69-72.

Bibliography

Awad EA: Interstitial myofibrositis: Hypothesis of the mechanism. Arch Phys Med 1973; 54:449-453.

Baker BA: The muscle trigger: Evidence of overload injury. Journal of Neurology and Orthopaedic Medicine and Surgery 1986; 7:35-43.

Barnes JF: Five years of myofascial release. Physical Therapy Forum (mid-atlantic edition) September 16, 1987.

Barnes JF: Therapeutic insight: Orthopaedics and sports medicine. Physical Therapy Forum May 13, 1987.

Barnes JF: Therapeutic insight: Sports and optimum performance. Physical Therapy Forum April 15, 1987.

Barnes JF: Therapeutic insight: The body is a self correcting mechanism. Physical Therapy Forum July 8, 1987.

Barnes JF: Therapeutic insight: "You will just have to live with it!" Physical Therapy Forum (Atlantic Edition) September 24, 1986.

Bartoli V, Dorigo B, Grissillo D, et al: Fibrositic myofascial pain in intermittent claudication: Significance of trigger areas in the calf. Angiology 1980; 31:11-20.

Bengtsson A, Henriksson KG, Jorfeldt L et al: Primary fibromyalgia, a clinical and laboratory study of 55 patients. Scand J Rheumatol 1986; 29:817-821.

Bengtsson A, Henriksson KG, Larson J. Muscle biopsy in primary fibromyalgia. Scand J Rheumatol 1986; 15:1-6.

Bennet RM: The fibrositis/fibromyalgia syndrome: Current issues and prospectives. Am J Med 1986; 81(supp 3a):43-49.

Benoit P, Belt WD: Some effects of local anesthetic agents on skeletal muscle. Exp Neurol 1972; 34:264-278.

Bourne IHJ: Treatment of painful conditions of the abdominal wall with local injections. Practitioner 1980; 224:921-925.

Brooke RI, Stenn PG: Postinjury myofascial pain dysfunction syndrome: Its etiology and prognosis. Oral Surgery 1978; 45:846-850.

Brooke RI, Stenn PG, Mothersill KJ: The diagnosis and conservative treatment of myofascial pain dysfunction syndrome. Oral Medicine 1977; 44:844-852.

Brown T, Nemiah JC, Barr, JS, et al: Psychologic factors in low-back pain. N Eng J Med 1954; 251:123-128.

Bunch RW: Appeal to intelligence and common sense. Physical Therapy Bulletin May 11, 1988.

Bunch RW: Myofascial release traced back decades. Physical Therapy Bulletin February 17, 1988.

Cheney FD: Muscle tenderness in 100 consecutive psychiatric patients. Diseases of the Nervous Systems 1969; 30:478-481.

Cohen SR: Follow-up evaluation of 105 patients with myofascial pain-dysfunction syndrome. J Am Den Assoc 1978; 97:825-828.

Cooper AL: Trigger-point injection: Its place in physical medicine. Arch Phys Med Rehabil 1961; Oct:704-709.

Cooper BC, Alleva M, Cooper DL, et al: Myofascial pain dysfunction: Analysis of 476 patients. Laryngoscope 1986; 96:1099-1106.

Crockett DJ, Foreman ME, Alden L, et al: A comparison of treatment modes in the management of myofascial pain dysfunction syndrome. Biofeedback and Self-Regulation 1986; 11:279-291.

Cubelli R, Caselli M, Neri M: Pain endurance in unilateral cerebral lesions. Cortex 1984; 20:369-375.

Danneskiold-Samsoe B, Christiansen E, Andersen RB: Myofascial pain and the role of myoglobin. Scand J Rheumatol 1986; 15:154-178.

DeJong RH: Defining pain terms. JAMA 1980; 244:143.

Dorigo B, Bartoli V, Grissillo D, et al: Fibrositic myofascial pain in intermittent claudication. Effect of anesthetic block of trigger points on exercise tolerance. Pain 1979; 6:183-190.

Dorko B: Craniosacral therapy and reason. Physical Therapy Bulletin March 9, 1988. p 5.

Dweck J: Anger blocked by fear. Energy and Character 1980; 7:32-40.

Engel GL: "Psychogenic" pain and the pain-prone patient. Am J Med 1959; 26:899-918.

Esposito CJ, Veal SJ, Farman AG: Alleviation of myofascial pain with ultrasonic therapy. J Prosthet Dent 1984; 51:106-108.

Feldenkrais M: Awareness Through Movement. New York, Harper & Row, Publishers, 1977.

Fell L: Freedom from myofascial dysfunction. Physical Therapy Forum (atlantic edition) October 29, 1986; vol 5:1, 4.

Fischer AA: The present status of neuromuscular thermography. Postgrad Med 1986; special number 79:26-33.

Fischer AA: Pressure threshold meter: Its use for quantification of tender spots. Arch Phys Med Rehabil 1986; 67:836-838.

Fischer AA: Letter to the editor. Pain 1987; 28:411-414.

Fordyce WE: A behavioral perspective on chronic pain. Br J Clin Psychol 1982; 21:313-320.

Frykholm R: Cervical nerve root compression resulting from disc degeneration and root-sleeve fibrosis. Act Chir Scand 1951; 160(supp):158-159.

Gassler JH: If it works, it's for different reasons. Physical Therapy Bulletin April 27, 1988; Vol 3: p 7.

Goddard MD, Reid JD: Movements induced by straight leg raising in the lumbo-sacral roots, nerves and plexus, and in the intrapelvic section of the sciatic nerve. J Neurol Neurosurg Psychiatry 1965; 28:12-17.

Gunn CC: Type IV acupuncture points. American Journal of Acupuncture 1977; 5:51-52.

Hall R: Barnes' theory, marketing style questioned. Physical Therapy Bulletin March 23, 1988; vol 3: p 5.

Hecaen H, Albert M: Human Neuropsychology. New York, Wiley, 1978.

Hubbell SL, Thomas M: Postpartum cervical myofascial pain syndrome: Review of four patients. Obstet Gynecol 1985; 65(supp 3):565-575.

Hunter C: Myalgia of the abdominal wall. Can Med Assoc J 1983; Feb:157-161.

Ignelzi RJ, Atkinson JH: Pain and its modulation. Part 1. Afferent mechanisms. Neurosurgery 1980; 6:577-583.

Ignelzi RJ, Atkinson JH: Pain and its modulation. Part 2. Efferent mechanisms. Neurosurgery 1980; 6:584-590.

Kellgren JH: Deep pain sensibility. Lancet 1949; June:943-949.

Kellgren JH: Observations on referral pain arising from muscle. Clin Sci, 1939; 3:175-190.

Kelly M: Lumbago and abdominal pain. Med J Aust 1942; 1:311-317.

Kielinski A: Myofascial release adds dimension to PT's private practice. Physical Therapy Forum January 18, 1984; vol 3: p 1, 6.

Kraft GH, Johnson EW, LaBan MM: The fibrositis syndrome. Arch Phys Med Rehabil 1968; 49:155-162.

Krout RR: Trigger points. J Am Podiatr Med Assoc 1987; 77:269.

Laskin DM, Block S: Diagnosis and treatment of myofascial pain-dysfunction (MPD) syndrome. J Prosthet Dent 1986; 56:75-84.

Lethem JPD, Salde, JDG, Troup, et al: Outline of a fear-avoidance model of exaggerated pain perception. Behav Res Ther 1983; 21:401-408.

Lewit K: The needle effect in the relief of myofascial pain. Pain 1979; 6:83-90.

Long C II: Myofascial pain syndromes. Part I -General characteristics and treatment. Henry Ford Hosp Med Bulletin 1956; 4:189-192.

Long C II: Myofascial pain syndromes. Part II -Syndromes of the head, neck and shoulder girdle. Henry Ford Hosp Med Bulletin 1955; 3:22-28.

Mance D, McConnell B, Ryan PA, et al: Myofascial pain syndrome. J Am Podiatr Med Assoc 1986; 76:328-331.

Melnick J: Trigger areas and refractory pain in duodenal ulcer. NY State J Med 1957; 57:1073-1076.

Melzack R: Myofascial trigger points: Relation to acupuncture and mechanisms of pain. Arch Phys Med Rehabil 1981; 62:114-117.

Miller J: There is no comparison since myofascial release. Physical Therapy Forum July 8, 1987; vol 6, no 27: p 1-2.

Miller B, Not the trademark but the arrogance involved. Physical Therapy Bulletin, January 13, 1988, 3:5.

Murray GR, Durh, DCL: Myofibrositis as a simulator of other maladies. Lancet 1929; January:113-116.

Nel H: Myofascial pain-dysfunction syndrome. J Prosthet Dent 1978; 40:438-441.

Perl ER: Sensitization of nociceptors and its relation to sensation, in: Bonica JJ, Albe-Fessard D (eds): Advances in Pain Research and Therapy. New York, Raven Press, 1976, Vol 1.

Perl ER: Unraveling the story of pain, in: Fields, HL (ed): Advances in Pain Research and Therapy. New York, Raven Press, 1985, Vol 9.

Price DD, Harkins SW, Baker C: Sensory-affective relationships among different types of clinical and experimental pain. Pain 1987; 28:297-307.

Reeves JL, Jaeger B, Graff-Radford SB: Reliability of the pressure algometer as a measure of myofascial trigger point sensitivity. Pain 1986; 24:313-321.

Reynolds MD: The development of the concept of fibrositis. J Hist Med Allied Sci 1983; 38:5-35.

Reynolds MD: Myofascial trigger point syndromes in the practice of rheumatology. Arch Phys Med Rehabil 1981; 62:111-14.

Rowe CS: Myofascial release and craniosacral therapy—A personal experience. Physical Therapy Forum September 27, 1986.

Shpuntoff H: Biofeedback electromyography and inhibition release in myofascial pain dysfunction cases. NY J Dent 1977; 47:304-309.

Simons DG: Myofascial trigger points: A need for understanding. Arch Phys Med Rehabil 1981; 62:97-99.

Simons DG: Myofascial pain syndromes due to trigger points: 1. Principles, diagnosis, and perceptuating factors. Manual Medicine 1985; 1:67-71.

Simons DG: Myofascial pain syndromes due to trigger points: 2. Treatment and single-muscle syndromes. Manual Medicine 1985; 1:72-77.

Simons DG, Travell JG: Myofascial trigger points: A possible explanation. Pain 1981; 10:106-109.

Sjaastad O, Saunte C, Graham JR: Chronic paroxysmal hemicrania. VII. Mechanical precipitation of attacks: New cases and localization of trigger points. Cephalogia 1984; 4:113-118.

Sola AE: Treatment of myofascial pain syndromes, in Benedetti C (ed): Advances in Pain Research and Therapy New York, Raven Press, 1984, Vol 7.

Sola AE: Trigger point therapy, in Roberts JR, Hedges JR (eds): Clinical Procedures in Emergency Medicine Philadelphia, WB Saunders, 1985.

Sola AE, Rodenberg ML, Gettys BB: Incidence of hypersensitive areas in posterior shoulder muscles. Am J Phys Med 1955; 34:585-590.

Sola AE, Williams RL: Myofascial pain syndromes. Neurology, 1956; 6:91-95.

Styf J, Lysell E: Chronic compartment syndrome in erector spinae muscle. Spine 1987; 12:680-682.

Talaat AM, El-Dibany, MM, El-Garf A: Physical therapy in the management of myofascial pain dysfunction syndrome. Ann Otol Rhinol Laryngol 1986; 95:225-228.

Taylor TC: Myofascial release techniques. Physical Therapy Forum June 4, 1986; 23:1-3.

Torebjork HE, Ocho, JL, Shady W: Referred pain from intraneural stimulation of muscle fascicles in the median nerve. Pain 1984; 18:145-156.

Travell JG: Myofascial trigger points: clinical view in: Bonica JJ, Albe-Fessard, D (eds): Advances in Pain Research and Therapy New York, Raven Press, 1976, Vol 1.

Trott PH, Gross AN: Physiotherapy in diagnosis and treatment of myofascial pain dysfunction syndrome. Int J Oral Surg 1978; 7:360-365.

Troup JDG, Slade PD: Fear avoidance and chronic musculoskeletal pain. Stress Medicine 1985; 1:217-220.

Upledger JE: Bunch challenged on several points, Physical Therapy Bulletin 3(12):5. March 30, 1988.

Webber TD: Diagnosis and modification of headache and shoulder-arm-hand syndrome. J Am Osteopath Assoc 1973;72:697-710.

Weinstein G: The diagnosis of trigger points by thermography. Academy of Neuro-muscular Thermography: Clinical Proceedings, Postgraduate Medicine. Custom Communications, 1986.

Wolfe F: The clinical syndrome of fibrositis. AM J Med 1986; 81(Suppl 3A):7-14.

Wolfe F, Cathey MA: Prevalence of primary and secondary fibrositis. J Rheumatol 1983; 10:965-968.

Wolff BB, Langley S: Cultural factors and the response to pain: A review. American Anthropologist 1968; 70:494-501.

Zohn DA: The quadratus lumborum: An unrecognized source of back pain, clinical and thermographic aspects. Orthopaedic Review 1985; 15:87-92.

Index